Our Brains at War

Our Brains at War

The Neuroscience of Conflict and Peacebuilding

MARI FITZDUFF

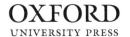

OXFORD
UNIVERSITY PRESS

OXFORD

UNIVERSITY PRESS

Oxford University Press is a department of the University of Oxford. It furthers
the University's objective of excellence in research, scholarship, and education
by publishing worldwide. Oxford is a registered trade mark of Oxford University
Press in the UK and certain other countries.

Published in the United States of America by Oxford University Press
198 Madison Avenue, New York, NY 10016, United States of America.

Library of Congress Cataloging-in-Publication Data
Names: Fitzduff, Mari, author.
Title: Our brains at war : the neuroscience of conflict and peacebuilding /
by Mari Fitzduff.
Description: New York, NY : Oxford University Press, 2021. |
Includes bibliographical references and index.
Identifiers: LCCN 2020053467 (print) | LCCN 2020053468 (ebook) |
ISBN 9780197512654 (hardback) | ISBN 9780197512678 (epub) |
ISBN 9780197512685
Subjects: LCSH: Social conflict—Psychological aspects. |
Conflict management—Psychological aspects. |
Peace-building—Psychological aspects. | War—Psychological aspects.
Classification: LCC HM1121 .F58 2021 (print) | LCC HM1121 (ebook) |
DDC 303.6—dc23
LC record available at https://lccn.loc.gov/2020053467
LC ebook record available at https://lccn.loc.gov/2020053468

DOI: 10.1093/oso/9780197512654.001.0001

To Iseult and Ellie, who are our future

Contents

Preface

It was an October evening in Belfast. The war had been dragging on for over twenty years, with no end in sight. My office in the city center was still being shaken by bombs on a regular basis: it was just around the corner from the Europa Hotel, known as the most bombed hotel in the world, which had suffered thirty-six bomb attacks during the so-called Troubles—the euphemism for the conflict in Northern Ireland. I was making my way up to the university area when my car suddenly died at the top of a street called Sandy Row, where shootings and bombings were a frequent occurrence. It was a staunchly loyalist area of Belfast and a traditional heartland for the paramilitary Ulster Defence Association. The Ulster Defence Association was using violence to keep Northern Ireland within the United Kingdom, as opposed to the violence of the Irish Republican Army (IRA), which was being used to try to force a politically united island of Ireland. Car maintenance not being my forte, I duly went into a pub, looked helpless (apologies to my feminist friends), and immediately was surrounded by a group of burly men, who offered to help. When I explained I was on my way to the nearby Queen's University, they suggested I give them my keys and they would sort out the car while I was away. I gave them the keys, and on my walk up to the university I wondered where else in the world you would freely give the key of your car to the patrons of a pub that was a known lair for paramilitaries—and know it would be OK—and this despite my accent being from the South of Ireland, which was the purported enemy of such men? A few hours later, I returned. The men told me they had taken the car to the garage of a friend, and he had fixed it, and it was grand now—"grand" being a shorthand term in Northern Ireland for all being OK. I offered to buy a round of drinks, but they refused and sent me on my way with their good wishes.

A few weeks later, the same car had a puncture and came to an abrupt stop opposite the office of Sinn Féin, the political wing of the IRA, who were the enemies of the loyalists. There were a group of men—"heavies," as we called bodyguards—outside the office, which was the lair of Gerry Adams, the leader of Sinn Féin. I stepped out of the car, put my hands in the air in supplication—and the whole group came over to the car, lifted it between them without the need for a lever, put on my spare tire, and sent me on my way with their good wishes. Once again, there was a contrast between what I know of how such men treated their out-group enemies—the British and the loyalists—and the ordinary decency that is actually the hallmark of most communities and people in Northern Ireland.

Living as I had in what were called "the Killing Fields" of Co. Tyrone—so called because it had the highest rate of killings in Northern Ireland outside of one Belfast zone—I had marveled over the years at how many of the people (almost always men) involved in IRA activities in our area were the same ones who helped the grannies get their groceries, coached the children in the neighborhood football club, attended church services on a Sunday, and even did the church collections. And I wondered how these men compartmentalized their actions, reserving all their goodness for their own communities and having no qualms about murdering their enemies on the other side. How did they (and the many other paramilitaries and their communities that I subsequently met from other countries) tell their histories to themselves so that they were always the victims and the other side, always the aggressors, often with complete disregard for many proven facts? How was it that their deadly deeds, which injured and maimed not just men but also women and children—wedding parties, football watchers, pub-loads of drinkers—were always justified by them, but others' similar deeds were never justified? What was it that so energized social grievances, or political or religious ideologies, in such a fundamentalist way, leading to so many being prepared not just to kill others but often to risk their own death while out on their killing sprees or through prison hunger strikes? Why were so many people willing to kill or be killed over a cartoon, a flag, a piece of clothing, a book, or a song? Why were historical memories about enemies so long—often about events that had happened hundreds or, in some cases, thousands of years ago? Were toxic leaders at fault or psychopathic personalities who were prone to use violence? Are conflicts always the product of unjust social and economic systems or the product of groups who feel themselves to have a distinctive ethnic, cultural, or religious identity that they perceive is disrespected and threatened? And—perhaps the biggest question of all—are violence and war, which appear to be so ubiquitous, "natural" to humankind and, if so, why?

An even more disturbing thought was that while we assume war and conflict are repugnant to most human beings, is this actually true? A gentle and intelligent professor and prime minister from the Republic of Ireland once said to me, "Of course everyone wants peace, don't they Mari?" It made me stop and wonder. As part of my doctoral studies I had interviewed many paramilitaries from both sides of the war in Northern Ireland, and almost all said that they had never felt more "alive" than while out on what they called "a night of action" (i.e., their killing missions for what they saw as their communities).

So many questions—few of which seemed to be answered in the political or international relations textbooks that I initially studied, which are still the normal tools used by many academics and policymakers trying to gain an understanding of today's wars. Living with my family in what was a war zone, with helicopters continually overhead, armed soldiers frequently patrolling our country roads, republican and loyalist murders happening with a few miles of our home, my husband's family business blown up, our local post office—run by his aunt—robbed so many times it had to close, I felt compelled to try to understand what was happening, and why, and to wonder what could be done to change it.

My first foray into the field of "conflict resolution," as it was then called, came in the mid-1980s when I ventured into a newly developing professional field—that of mediation. So new was it that when I started to teach it in the local university, about half the class who came thought it was about meditation! Eventually, it resulted in the setting up, with some colleagues, of an organization called the Mediation Network. This became the main providing agency for mediators for street conflicts in Northern Ireland, as well as mediators who worked on many shuttle and face-to-face mediations between paramilitaries, political parties, communities, and governments in Northern Ireland and subsequently on many international conflicts. Given that such discussions were always fraught with difficulties, I also produced a group skills book suggesting over a hundred ways of having productive discussions about issues of justice, equity, symbols, emotions, history, community conflicts, etc., a generic version of which is in use in many conflicts around the world today (Fitzduff and Williams, 2019).

My main intellectual interest was in trying to understand why some people in Northern Ireland who had initially chosen to use violence to address the conflict, some of whom had been jailed, eventually abandoned such a strategy in favor of dialogue efforts, and this question became the focus for my doctoral work. Somewhat to my surprise, I discovered that very few of these people had been talked or reasoned out of their support for violence. By far the majority who had changed were those whose minds and behaviors had been transformed through experiences that had subsequently created emotional and instinctual challenges for them. I was also very interested to hear how lonely many of their lives were, given that they had moved out of their belief or action "tribes," and there were few alternative institutes or political parties to support them in their choices. Even more important, I was struck by the problems these findings posed for current efforts to increase intergroup understanding between warring communities, as almost all of our existing change programs in Northern Ireland were focused on a belief in the use of contact, argument, and reasoning between groups in the hope of changing attitudes and, even more important, behavior.

I was soon to get a chance to test such strategies. Following my PhD research, in 1990, I was appointed as the first chief executive of a body set up to begin to fund both policy and practice conflict resolution efforts in Northern Ireland. This was the Community Relations Council, which became the main body for subsequent funding policy and community reconciliation work in Northern Ireland.[1] It was a recipient of extensive funds from both the European Union and the British government. Although such work, and through my subsequent international research, consultancy, and mediation work as the Director of UNU/INCORE, a United Nations University Center, I came again and again to appreciate how little part reason often plays in social conflicts—and how much is played by instincts and emotions.

My more recent work as the founding director, in Brandeis University, of a graduate program for professionals involved in over seventy conflicts around the world not only confirmed such a judgment, but also gave me a chance to develop a learning program, in conjunction with the program participants, that would augment existing international relations approaches to conflict. This new program was based on learning from the existing fields of the social sciences, particularly social psychology, as well as the emerging fields of the biosocial sciences, which became an interdisciplinary field devoted to understanding how biological systems can affect social processes and behavior. Such an approach takes heart and wisdom from the advent of the behavioral sciences—in particular, the field of social neuroscience, which studies the effects of psychological, neurological, emotional, cultural, and social factors, as well as cognitive factors, and their effect on human decision-making in various fields.

The advent of behavioral economics has revolutionized the field of economics, involving efforts to incorporate more realistic notions of human

---

[1] https://www.community-relations.org.uk/

nature into economics and ways of looking at decisions other than those implied by classical theories of economics. Governments too are now utilizing these new behavioral approaches for public policy strategies; for example, the UK government has set up a "Nudge" unit based on behavioral neuroscience to help shape public policy, as has the Australian government. Social media companies such as Google, Facebook, and Twitter are (rightly or wrongly—see Chapter 9 of this volume) using neuromarketing as part of their business strategies. The World Bank is increasingly turning to the behavioral sciences to help tackle seemingly intractable social and economic challenges such as the faster facilitation of development in many parts of the world. Many of these companies are working on the assumption that drawing on insights from behavioral sciences and, in particular, the social neurosciences can generate new kinds of interventions that can be successful and profitable for the business communities and/or cost-effective for policymakers. The development of such approaches has in recent decades been assisted by the advent of new technologies such as functional magnetic resonance imaging and hormonal and genetic testing, which have either validated or enhanced our understanding about previously little understood social factors that shape our relationships with each other, both individually and collectively in groups.

As yet the field of conflict resolution—now more often called peacebuilding—has been little affected by such new strategies. We see almost nothing about such an interdisciplinary approach in our textbooks for peacebuilders or for today's soldiers whose military responsibilities are in many cases being refocused on conflict prevention, as well as community and institutional development in conflicted and post-conflict societies. We need to understand that we as humans everywhere are affected by the many predisposed body/brain legacy patterns that hamper our work and of which we are often unaware. The problem is that if left unnoted and unattended, such tendencies will hinder our capacities to live together and to resolve our differences without the use of violence. This book sets out to address these missing factors.

Caveats

A knowledge of the social and biosocial psychological sciences is important to the effectiveness of the conflict resolution and peacebuilding field, but we need to be careful to recognize their limitations as tools for understanding conflict and effecting more peaceful societies.

The number one limitation is the fact that most of the research outlined in this book has been conducted by and on what are called WEIRD people (i.e., Western, educated, industrialized, rich, and democratic; Henrich, Heine, and Norenzayan, 2010). Thus far, WEIRD populations have been vastly overrepresented in social psychological research. By studying only such populations, researchers often fail to take account of the diversity of the global population, and thus applying the findings from WEIRD populations only can hinder the relevance of the research. While this book has tried to take as wide an approach to global research as is possible (see Chapter 7 of this volume), it has, like my previous books on global conflict (Fitzduff and Stout, 2006), been limited by the research capacity of many universities around the world, whose meager finances have made it very difficult for them to free up their academics to undertake the kind of research that is needed to supplement this book.

The fact is that *structural and societal contexts* that are unfair and potentially humiliating to certain groups are often the main facilitators of conflicted and violent behavior between groups (Stewart, 2008). Wars start primarily not because of biosocial factors but because such factors come into play through manipulation and violence within a situation where people of particular identities feel unequal and excluded. Most of our recent wars have come about because of issues of inequality or exclusion. Given that unfairness is actually physically felt (Chapter 3 of this volume), it is logical to believe that if such contexts had been handled differently, then individual and group differences might just be part of the normal grist of a society that is well-informed regarding the need to manage diverse groups. Approaches using only psychocultural/sociocultural understandings can only be effective in the long term if structural issues are addressed.

The third caveat is the fact that, as the book clearly outlines, not all human brains are the same: for example, some people tend more easily to be suspicious of others, and some are more open to new people and new experiences. These differences clearly cross race and ethnic lines and cannot be used to justify the legacy of scientific racism—that is, the use of scientific techniques and hypotheses to support or justify presumptions of racial inferiority or superiority, which, although not often spoken about publicly now, are in some quarters still with us.

None of the research in this book will give ballast to anyone interested in eliciting such differences for reasons of discrimination. Alas, the contrary is true—we are all of us, of whatever part of the world, or whatever part of our group or nations indicted for the emotional and cognitive confusions that we often bring to bear on the situations in which we live, work, and make war and, sometimes, peace.

My fourth caveat is that we also need to know that there is nothing determinist about what is revealed by our genetic or hormonal testing or our magnetic resonance imaging scans. While our genes, brains, and hormones can predispose us to certain ideas, they are not predestined: brains can be relatively plastic, and our biopsychological and genetic tendencies can be altered (somewhat) by our environments. *Predisposition does not mean predetermination.* There is no individual or group that cannot change their behavior toward another individual or group. While the research suggests that predisposed characteristics can be relatively hard to change, it also notes that such change, if carefully managed, is possible.

What such different strategies might be and how they may add to the effectiveness of peacebuilding—which I define as the capacity of a society to solve its conflicts through political, legal, or dialogue processes, rather than through violence—can hopefully be elucidated by the knowledge in this book.

Introduction

The certainty with which we act now might seem ghastly not only to
future generations but to our future selves as well.
                                              —Sapolsky (2017, p. 674)

The Future of Conflict

This book is being written at a time when the failures of the Western
interventions into Iraq and Afghanistan and the fragmentation of Syria into
thousands of militias of various hues, with ever-changing interventions by
at least seven other countries, have laid bare the limitations of traditional
war methodologies. While the wars in Afghanistan and Iraq did stimulate
some debates about the limitations of traditional approaches to war (Debs
and Monteiro, 2014), such limitations have yet to be taken into account by
many policymakers, national leaders, and academics. As I write, the United
States, under the guidance of a relatively new president, is once again putting its hopes into newer, better, and more expensive war equipment to protect itself without any clear indication of how this can contribute to a more
peaceful world or even to a safer US society. Such a strategy neglects to note
that nineteen amateur plane hijackers, with the threat of no more than box-
cutter knives, ended any idea of a "safe" society in the United States or elsewhere on September 11, 2001.

The continuing development of smaller technologies also belies the whole-
sale purchase of billion-dollar armaments. For example, in October 2019, it
was revealed that just eighteen drones and seven cruise missiles—all cheap
and unsophisticated compared to modern military aircraft—disabled half of
Saudi Arabia's crude oil production. They destroyed 5 percent of the world's
oil supplies and raised the world price of oil by 20 percent.

An overriding belief in primarily using military force to solve conflicts was
challenged in an open letter by over 120 former US three- and four-star generals to the US House and Senate leadership in 2017. The letter called on them

Our Brains at War. Mari Fitzduff, Oxford University Press (2021). © Oxford University Press.
DOI: 10.1093/oso/9780197512654.003.0001

not to expand the military budget at the expense of soft-power approaches, and to "ensure that resources for the International Affairs Budget [which funds diplomacy, developmental and peacebuilding efforts] keep pace with the growing global threats and opportunities we face."[1] The signatories included General David Petraeus, a former CIA director and a retired admiral, and James Stavridis, the former NATO supreme allied commander (Cahn, 2016). This point had previously been implicitly made by former General Petraeus in his guidelines for the army in Afghanistan, which emphasized the practice of soft power, even by the military (ISAF Public Affairs Office, 2010). A decade previously former UK General Sir Rupert Smith also emphasized the importance and the priority of power other than military power (R. Smith, 2005).[2] Smith concludes that while confrontations and conflicts

> exist all around the world, and states still have armed forces, which they use as symbols of power . . . war as cognitively known to most noncombatants, war as battle in a field between men and machinery, war as a massive deciding event in a dispute in international affairs, industrial war—such war no longer exists. We now are engaged, constantly and in many permutations, in *war amongst the people*. We must adapt our approach and organize our institutions to this overwhelming reality. (https://www.historynet.com/interview-rupert-smith-cant-win-war-terror.htm; emphasis added)

Smith had been Deputy Supreme Commander of the Allied Powers Europe from 1998 to 2001, and much of his experience came from the conflicts in the former Yugoslavia and in Northern Ireland. Having worked alongside all parties in Northern Ireland, including the military and the police, I was aware that the best of the British Army, as well as the police and the British and Irish governments, were often at a loss about how best to contain and eliminate a few hundred IRA and loyalist bombers and gunmen, despite the presence of over forty thousand people in the security forces. These were the "war among the people" wars that Smith referred to—and in these and other intra-societal wars, which are most of the wars today, the best and most expensive munition weapons are often useless.

Most of the wars I will be talking about in this book are what Kaldor (2012) called the "new wars"—that is, those that are mainly fought within countries,

---

[1] https://www.usglc.org/downloads/2017/02/FY18_International_Affairs_Budget_House_Senate.pdf

[2] https://www.historynet.com/interview-rupert-smith-cant-win-war-terror.htm

or initially within countries, and often by non-state actors as opposed to state military forces. Such wars are often supported by a wider community of nations whose interests are engaged by them, which often act as proxy stakeholders. These new wars are particularly difficult to understand using traditional approaches to international political frameworks. Unfortunately, most of the much-needed research on today's conflicts is usually undertaken by academics, many of whom fail to appreciate, understand, or even accept the seemingly irrational logic of many of these new wars. Most political and international relations scholars have previously assumed that nation-states are the principal actor in international relations, and their prime focus of study has been on inter-state relationships. Their work usually implies that the decision makers are state rational actors who will always choose to pursue the national interest.

> The conception of the world offered by realists is easy to grasp. Rational, calculating, and egoistic states are the most important actors in a non-hierarchical international system. States' survival strategies are based on amassing power and forming alliances against any state that threatens to upset the existing balance of power. Realists also believe that the security dilemma can be limited by a balance of power. Power politics is the name of the game and the game is zero-sum. That is, one state's gain is another state's loss. (Al-Rodham, 2013)

However, although internal wars can become international state proxy wars, most of the threats that states face come from their own non-state actors and illegal paramilitaries who are often fighting for the power of the state itself—or for the power of a transnational or transglobal identity. Unfortunately, international relations researchers often fail to appreciate, or indeed to have the vocabulary to deal with, the instinctual and emotional factors involved in such conflicts despite the fact that they are probably the most dominant factor in many of the identity wars of today.

Even in the Western world a major national/state decision, the Brexit referendum, was seen by many critics to be dominated "not by sober analysis and evidence-based reason, but by hysteria, hatred, savage emotions, and the sinister monster of exclusionary, ethnic nationalism" (Foster, 2016). In the United States, the widespread disbelief and confusion around the 2016 election of President Donald Trump as president was only possible because of a misunderstanding by many analysts that political behavior, for the most part, is rational. Unfortunately, they failed to realize that in many cases our political and leadership choices are driven by value predispositions such as perceived loss of identity and a context of threat and exclusion (Fitzduff, 2017). In both the Brexit and Trump campaigns, leaders used their rhetoric not to appeal rationally to followers' interests but to appeal emotionally to their instinctual and emotional predispositions, which in turn became the basis of widespread decision-making (Grillo, 2017). In many other countries today people are voluntarily electing right-wing political parties to govern them or choosing autocrats as their leaders. Unfortunately, the perceptions of threats today, particularly those incurred by increasing globalization, migration, and inequalities, can be all too easily mobilized by political and military leadership, and the "othering" of individuals or groups—that is, emphasizing a person or group of people as intrinsically different from oneself—can follow all too easily and significantly escalate a conflict.

Fortunately, the mismatch between wars as they are and wars as many soldiers, politicians, and presidents would like them to be is increasingly understood by those at the sharpest and most authoritative level of the military. It has led to an ever-growing number of military colleges opening their doors to the profession and the skills of peacebuilding and an increase in the number of professional and academic peacebuilders working in these colleges. The author and many of her colleagues are frequent faculty members for war colleges such as West Point, the US Army War College in Carlisle, Marine Special Operations in Tampa, the Army and Navy Academy in San Diego, the National Defense University, and the Inter-American Defense College. Many peacebuilding graduate programs, such as those at George Mason and Brandeis universities, welcome military forces. Sandhurst—the prime officers' college in the United Kingdom—has also been inviting professional and academic peacebuilders to partner with its military faculty to increase the skills of their officers in exploring alternatives to the use of force for resolving conflicts in the field. Although still minor in relation to war colleges, the professional field of conflict resolution/peacebuilding is growing fast. When I established our international graduate professional program at Brandeis in 2004, there were only ten such graduate programs in the world addressing conflict resolution/peacebuilding strategies. At latest count there are over 160 graduate programs around the world addressing these issues.

Vital to these programs is an additional understanding of the realities of our biosocial and neural legacies and the way they affect the development and maintenance of war. Such an understanding may help us to work more realistically, more compassionately, and more effectively with conflicted groups whose behavior is often dictated to, and limited by, human social and physical processes whose consequences we are only just beginning to understand and appreciate. Being aware of how our minds and bodies work to affect our social and group behavior to other groups is critically important. Asghar (2016) has suggested,

> The point of acknowledging the thorny aspects of human nature and our similarities to the animal world isn't to make us grow fatalistic. . . . I believe it's our highest duty as human beings. . . . I also believe that our ability to do so is impaired by when we don't look with absolute honesty at the unconscious forces and peculiar motivations that draw our fellow citizens to idols and icons. After all, condemning these fellow citizens as rubes and fools really won't bring about a better society.

In many ways, understanding these truths is both salutary and comforting, as a more thorough understanding of them can help us to shape our environments to avoid ignorantly supporting contexts that elicit the worst inclinations of our human predispositions.

The advent of technology that can actively track our brain and change our emotions, our ideas, and our choices by slight physical brain manipulations has been a humbling factor in our understanding of human nature (see Chapter 1 of this volume). Social psychology studies have long suggested many of the precise behaviors that are often elicited by particular contexts, and the latest findings in the neuroscience field have frequently confirmed their ideas. The advent of technology that can both read our brain and our bodies and assess their responses to particular contexts, even before we are conscious of them, is somewhat frightening. However, in the end I believe it is perhaps better to understand both our complexity and our predictability as individuals and social beings so that we can better ensure that we are not blindly led into situations by little-understood emotions and beliefs that often nudge us into conflictual and violent behavior toward many of our fellow citizens of this planet. My hope is that the contents of this book will enable us to base our strategies for peacebuilding on a more thorough understanding of the study of psychological and bio-physical correlates of social and political attitudes and behavior and more thoughtful approaches to our work than hitherto.

In undertaking this work I have tried to take a non-judgmental approach to the differences that seem to be evident between human beings and, for example, their genes, neural architecture, and hormones. As the research shows, people and groups *are* different in the way they think and process information, the kinds of emotions they bring to bear on decisions, the control they have over their emotions, the needs they have to belong to a group, what they prioritize as values, the importance of ideology in their lives, the way they identify enemies, the way they see facts, what they remember and forget, their fear and suspicions of out-groups, their need for leaders, etc. These differences are socially, biologically, and culturally influenced (see Chapter 7 of this volume) and are neither good nor bad. They just are—and they exist possibly because somewhere along the line such differences, and a mix of such differences, have been important for individual and group survival. What is important, I believe, is that we understand these differences and take them into account, and in my final chapter of this book I have made some suggestions as to how such insights can be usefully applied to the work of peacebuilding.

However, we also need to appreciate that much of the research about the recent findings of neuroscience is very tentative: many of the mechanisms used to measure such processes are still in their infancy, and some of their results are still quite fragile. The biosciences have been touted for their ability to look under the hood of our brains and perhaps to help us to see some of the mechanisms and processes that can create and perpetuate conflict. However, the reality is that many of the mechanisms used to measure such thoughts and behavior, such as functional magnetic resonance imaging, are still in their early stages and their results are often tentative. (In fairness, I have often found that the tentative nature of their findings is acknowledged by the researchers themselves.)

Perhaps it is best to approach these chapters with the usual caveat of Wikipedia—namely, "these sites are under construction." The social sciences and biosciences, and the partnerships between them, are currently very active disciplines, and I am aware that I may be giving the impression that there is far more consensus about many issues than is actually the case. I am also aware that by simplifying many explanations, particularly in the neuroscience field, I run the risk of underestimating their actual complexity and ignoring the relevance of such complexity to useful policy and practice. The book is, however, replete with references for further explorations by readers who can hopefully continue their interest into future insights than can be shared with both the military and peacebuilding fields.

Chapter 1: On Being Mortal

This chapter introduces people to the basics of what readers need to know about social psychology—that is, the study of how people's feelings, ideas and behaviors are influenced by the presence of others. It also looks at the increasingly important bio/neural factors such as genes, brain structure, and hormonal processes that are now being examined and understood as relevant to any study of human behavior, including group conflicts. In addition, it provides a brief introduction to the various methodologies that are increasingly able to measure social behavior, such as functional magnetic resonance imaging, electroencephalography, DNA analysis, and hormonal testing.

Chapter 2: The Amygdala Hijack

This chapter introduces the reader to the proven tenuous nature of reason when pitted against emotions. Contrary to what most of us believe, our human capacity for rational judgment is much (much!) shallower than we think, particularly in situations of conflict. The chapter will explain why social tensions can arise so easily and why murders, genocides, and mass killings can evolve so quickly in almost any situation. It looks at the tension between the parts of our brains that deal with our memories, pleasures, and fears and those that serve us through the use of analytic and logical reasoning. It also looks at how the balance between these varying parts of our brains can be different in different people and groups and how these differences can affect people's perspective on contentious issues such as immigration, military spending, and patriotism.

Chapter 3: Us and Others

This chapter looks at the importance of group belonging for feelings of safety and validation, particularly in times of conflict. It examines how and why varying group identities such as religion, ethnicity, and social and cultural identities enable people to deny the importance of the lives of members of other groups, or even their own lives. It looks at the social and biological advantages of group membership, which can increase our suspicion and rejection of others. It also looks at how we usually understand others not by thinking but by feeling and addresses the role of mirror neurons in this process, as well as hormones such as oxytocin, and their implications for group conflict. It considers the phenomenon of emotional contagion between groups, which will drive them to group behavior that can be contrary to their "normal" behavior.

Chapter 4: My Truth or Your Truth?

This chapter looks at the nature of beliefs and their relationship to "truth" or "facts." For many of us, far from our beliefs being "true," they are actually born out of a particular social context, allied to physiological needs such as a differing neural sensitivity to threats and the greater certainty of belief that a group can provide. Thus, beliefs are often what is termed "groupish" rather than necessarily true. The chapter examines why we often rationalize what our gut instincts tell us rather than care too much about fact-checking and why and how, once we form our beliefs, we have a tendency to see and find evidence to support them. It also looks at memories (including collective memories), which are also notoriously faulty—that is, our memories often reframe and edit events to create a story that suits what we need to believe today, rather than what is true.

Chapter 5: The Lure of Extremism

This chapter looks at the phenomenon of violent extremism or "terrorism"—so called depending on the context. It notes that fundamentalism (including violent fundamentalism) is a form of extreme belief—with the group aspects often more important than the actual beliefs. The chapter shows just how strongly our choices for membership of extreme groups are facilitated by our genetic, neurological, and hormonal predispositions to situations of tension and to danger, particularly when added to perceptions of group inequities and exclusion. It appears that membership of such groups is more often about a sense of solidarity and collectiveness than about truth, and strategies aimed at changing "beliefs" can have only a limited force. Thus, the actual as well as the expressed reasons for joining such groups need to be taken into account in designing strategies to change such memberships.

Chapter 6: Follow the Leader

This chapter looks at the importance of leaders in setting the tone and direction of contexts that are riven by confusion and conflict. The supremacy of emotions in choosing our leaders is particularly relevant in situations torn apart by conflict. In such situations our choices are often instinctual, dictated not only by our environment, our emotions, genetics, and brain structures but also by hormones such as adrenaline, norepinephrine, and cortisol, which inform our response to fear messages. This supremacy of emotions in choosing our leaders is particularly relevant in situations termed "weak psychological situations" such as crises or situations characterized by uncertainty, and by the presence and/or threat of out-groups. It appears that our desire for a strong leader who will provide us with security can often significantly outrank our desire for democracy and has important consequences for our capacity to manage conflict.

Chapter 7: Accultured Norms

This chapter looks at the importance of understanding the many cultural differences that exist between different groups and in different contexts around the world. Without a sensitivity to such differences, wars can be lost and positive influences minimized. These differences include the existence of high-context–low-context societies, differing hierarchical approaches to power and authority, collectivist versus individualist societies, differing emotion expression/recognition, gender differences, differing evidencing of empathy, face preferences, and communication styles. Lack of cultural attunement to these issues can exacerbate misunderstandings and conflicts, unless understood and factored into difficult strategies and dialogues.

Chapter 8: New Horizons, New Tribes

This chapter looks at the future of war in a world where social media are ubiquitous and at how our social and biological natures are affected, both for good and for evil, by their presence, particularly in times of conflict and war. Social media platforms such as Facebook and Twitter have already significantly changed how people, communities, and nations relate to each other, form new connections, or deepen older ones. They have also radically changed how people make judgments about leaders and other groups and how they act on those judgments. Such power is unprecedented and has potentially disastrous consequences if used in situations of tension and violence. It appears that our human social and biological tendencies make us easy prey for varied purveyors of conflict who wish to emotionally persuade us to support particular goals or objectives. We therefore need to find better ways to ensure that we can effectively prevent the hijacking of our human and emotional predispositions and that social media processes deliver on what is the best in our human biosocial nature and not the worst.

Chapter 9: The Next Adaptation?

This chapter looks at the research that shows that totally selfish behavior is the exception, not the rule. It examines the innate human tendencies and capacities that exist for cooperation between people, in contrast to the competitiveness that previous evolutionary psychology has suggested is the norm. However, the research is ambivalent about the future of such cooperation. It suggests that although socially and biologically humans have evolved for cooperation; so far it appears to be mainly with the people they perceive as their "own" group, and only gradually with other groups. The chapter looks at the question of whether we are asking too much of our biosocial histories that we should willingly expand our circles of concern to include the increasing refugee and migration movements that are changing the diverse nature of our societies. If we need to do this, how can it be done?

Chapter 10: Peacebuilding More Successfully?

This chapter addresses the suggestions that are emerging from the growing field of social behavioral psychology about how the work of peacebuilders, diplomats, armies, and others can use the insights noted in this book toward more effective peacebuilding efforts.

1

On Being Mortal

Evolution does not stop at the neck.

—Geher (2015)

Introduction

The violence Rwanda saw is nearly unimaginable. Between April and June 1994, it was estimated that between 500,000 and 1,000,000 Rwandans were killed over a period of one hundred days (Nowrojee, 1996). Machete- and club-wielding Hutus entered homes and slaughtered Tutsis, and some Hutus who had defended them, including children, women, and old people. These included many who had previously been their close neighbors and friends. The attackers burned down churches with hundreds or thousands of Tutsis inside—who had been betrayed by their priests. It was estimated that the killers, despite their primitive weapons, did their work five times as fast as the mechanized gas chambers used by the Nazis (Tiemessen, 2004). Sexual violence was also rife, with an estimated 250,000 to 500,000 women raped during the genocide (Nowrojee, 1996).

How could such atrocities happen? And how could this be just one among many other atrocities? In the former Yugoslavia war, how was it possible for a dozen drunken Serbian militiamen to raid a school gymnasium in which more than one hundred young Muslim women were being held with their infant children and gang-rape them over a period of twenty-six days, with some of the women being raped by as many as seven Serb militiamen (Fisk, 1993)? How did the regime of the Khmer Rouge under the leadership of Pol Pot, from 1975 to 1979, result in the deaths of approximately 1.5 to 2 million of its own people—nearly a quarter of Cambodia's 1975 population of 7.8 million (Heuveline, 2001)? How come that even today, people living with albinism—a genetic condition that causes white skin and hair—in Tanzania live in constant fear of being hunted like animals due to a brutal practice in

Our Brains at War. Mari Fitzduff, Oxford University Press (2021). © Oxford University Press.
DOI: 10.1093/oso/9780197512654.003.0002

which witchdoctors chop their limbs off and turn their butchered bodies into charms and potions (Drury, 2015; Velton, 2017).

What are the factors that led to these horrors, where neighbors turned to killing, often in horrific fashion, people whom they had lived alongside for decades? Is this human madness? Or, if not, what?

The question is one with which social psychologists and many others have struggled, particularly over the past few decades since the Holocaust. However, instead of thinking of such atrocities as being the problem of crazy individual madmen/madwomen, differing individual levels of innate aggression, or personal psychopathology, social psychologists look instead to the way people who are in groups behave toward one another. What makes apparently normal people, often with unbelievable speed, turn into the haters and killers of others and turn savagely against a group that is different than their own? Social psychologists, along with most of the rest of the world, were stunned by how Adolf Hitler could have produced such an extreme capacity for hate and cruelty in supposedly ordinary people. The Hitler regime was the most popular government in German history—in 1933, almost 40 percent of Germans voted for it ("Hitler Comes to Power," n.d.). The Nazi Party was not a small group who took over a country and committed the Holocaust of over six million against the wishes of its people. On the contrary, it had the support of huge numbers of people from across the social and political divides (Wilde, 2018). Similarly, after the massacres in Rwanda, the jails were crowded with over 130,000 prisoners accused of murder. How does a society descend to such barbarities?

In her reflections on the Holocaust, Hannah Arendt (1963) suggested a "banality of evil" perspective that rejects the notion that evil acts are the result of "sadistic monsters" and emphasizes that those who do such evil are usually ordinary people who find themselves in extraordinary circumstances.

Indeed, if we defined those who carry out such atrocities as being mad or psychopathic, it would mean we would have to redefine what it meant to be a "normal" human being. But perhaps we have to accept that carrying out such "inhumane" behavior is indeed a factor of "normal" humanness and that cruelty and violence can be elicited in most of us if certain group situations arise that stimulate it?

The study of just what such group situations are, and the tensions they often pose for normal people during conflicts and violence, has been an important part of social psychology for many years (Fitzduff and Stout, 2006). Such an approach does not deny, for example, the personality and influence of particular leaders on a conflict or the search for dominance of land or power by nations and groups. It does, however, suggest that an understanding of these factors is not enough without also understanding the social-psychological group needs that underpin people's and communities' responses to such tensions. In pursuit of such understanding, social psychologists have traditionally studied people's social behavior based on the collection and systematic analysis of observable and reported data. This includes studying people in their natural environments, in laboratory settings using complex and comparative experimental designs, and through field experiments, case studies, naturalistic observation, survey research, and nonconscious techniques such as priming their emotions through the use of flags and symbols.

Enter the Biosocial Sciences

The study of such issues by social psychologists has however been limited by the difficulty for researchers and others in managing the challenges thrown up by self-report methods, which are frequently subject to pressures to give socially acceptable responses, and the often unconscious limitations of bias on the part of subjects and of observers. Such limitations have challenged the field and, in some cases, have prevented it from being taken seriously. However, in the past decade or so, thanks to technological advancements that have assisted the growth of the biosciences, some of which use biological concepts and methods to inform and refine theories of social behavior, all of this has changed (Cacioppo and Decety, 2011).

This new focus on the social and psychological biosciences has assisted the development of many new fields such as neuropolitics, neurobiology, neuropsychology, genopolitics, political physiology, behavioral genetics, and cognitive neuroscience, all of which are investigating the interplay between the brain, society, and politics. Because of such developments, an increasing number of social psychology researchers are now integrating the study of biological markers of the brain or hormones or genes into their research to better understand processes that seem to be suggesting that our behaviors are influenced by biological factors of which we are often unaware. These studies have all helped to sharpen the field of traditional social psychology and in some cases validate many of its findings through biological processes that can be objectively measured; for example, it appears that many parts of our bodies and, in particular, our brains can be proven to play substantial roles in the facilitation of societal conflict (e.g., Tusche et al., 2013).

This research has been assisted by the advent of new technologies such as functional magnetic resonance imaging (fMRI), electroencephalography (EEG), and electrodermal activity (EDA) and by genetic and hormonal measuring techniques that have greatly enhanced our understanding of what is happening in our minds and bodies, often unknown to ourselves, as we live our daily lives (Doraiswamy, 2015). While many of these technological processes are at an early stage of development and are known for their tentative nature, they bring attention to the way in which our bodies and, particularly, our brains often autonomously and unconsciously affect our attitudes and behavior, and vice versa. The advent of technology that can actively track our brains and that change our emotions, our ideas, and our choices by slight physical brain changes or manipulations has been an enlightening and humbling factor in our understanding of human nature.

The Brain

These new genetics, brain, and hormonal sciences are providing very strong evidence that many of our personality traits, including how we relate to other groups, have at least some basis in the biology of the brain. The brain itself, which weighs about three pounds (1.4 kg), is built from approximately 100 billion nerve cells called neurons. Communication is effected by neurotransmitters, which transmit signals between nerve cells and other cells in the body. There are a 1,000 trillion synaptic connections between these 100 billion neurons, and these impulses transfer information through the cells in the brain regions, sometimes at a speed of 250 miles (400 km) per second. These chemical messengers can affect a wide variety of both physical and psychological functions in our bodies including our emotions, our appetites, our sleep, etc. They trigger our hormones such as serotonin, oxytocin, dopamine, cortisol, testosterone, estrogen, and adrenalin, which act directly on the body and influence our social interactions related to attention, communication, feelings, learning, memory, and recognition (Dfarhud et al., 2014). We can now trace which areas of our minds light up during different activities such as listening to music, problem-solving, mystical experiences, sexual excitement, and depression, as well as when we meet strangers, respond to apparent threats, etc. (Berridge and Kringelbach,

2015). Thanks to modern biochemistry and brain imagining, we can also proactively stimulate many of our emotions by specifically stimulating different areas of the brain (Selimbeyoglu and Parvizi, 2010; Volman et al., 2016), a practice that is increasingly used by social media platforms (see Chapter 8 of this volume).

Two regions of the brain are particularly important for people working in war and peacebuilding contexts to know about and to understand how they function. These are the part that processes our automatic/intuitive impulses (the amygdala) and the part that deals with our conscious/reasoned processes (the prefrontal cortex), although it needs to be remembered that there can be considerable interaction and overlap between the layers.

The *amygdala* is the size of an almond and is the part of our brain that deals with our senses, our memories, and our emotions, such as pleasure and fear. Its processes are automatic—sometimes called intuitive or implicit—and are impulsive or instinctive in nature, which means that we often have little choice about feeling them. This is the oldest part of our brain, reckoned to be at least 60 to 200 million years old. It records memories of behaviors that have produced feelings of good or bad experiences in our lifetimes and in those of our ancestors and is mainly responsible for our emotions. It exerts a very strong influence on our choices, often at an unconscious level, and particularly in fear-inducing situations of conflict. The amygdala can respond to stimuli that are too fleeting or faint for the thinking part of the brain—the cortex—to even note, and it is the driver of emotions and intuitive judgment within the brain. It is the alert button for any dangers on the horizon and for automatic and fast emotional responses that promote self and group preservation. These emotional reactions and understandings can be beneficial; for example, they can enable people to connect with others and thus increase their ability to protect the survival of an individual or group. However, they can also be harmful. The amygdala's prime focus is on possible threats to our well-being, and thus it is primed to respond and formulate reactions to possible individual or group fears. However, in doing so it can build up insecurity, fear, and divisive conflict between individuals and groups in many situations. Studies have also connected its reactive responses and judgments to emotions of morality, ideas of disgust, and ideals of perfection (Asp, Ramchandran, and Tranel, 2012), all of which can affect our responses to other groups: for example, individual differences in disgust sensitivity, as noted by increased amygdala functioning, were found to be predictive of implicit racial prejudice (Y. Liu et al., 2015).

The *prefrontal cortex* is the other extremely important section of the brain that is relevant to our peacebuilding focus. It concerns itself with conscious/rational processes. It is considered to be the "newer" brain and is deemed responsible for the development of human language, for abstract thought, for our imagination, for reasoning, and for our consciousness. It is intricately connected to the amygdala and influenced by it, and in return it tries to infuse amygdala instincts and emotions with secondary but often extremely important rational considerations. It is the part of the brain that searches already formed memories and contributes (or tries to contribute) a more analytic, logical, and thoughtful response to any situation.

Depending on the context, the amygdala or the cortex can come to the fore. Whenever we encounter a situation of possible danger and do not have time to think or delay our reactions, the amygdala, as our bodyguard, will literally trigger the hairs on the back of our necks even before our reasoning mind understands what is happening (Dickerson, 2015). It will also trigger our heart rate so that our muscles receive more blood and oxygen to prepare the body for physical action. And to further assist us, it will trigger the release of hormones such as adrenaline and cortisol, which gives us a quick surge of energy and diverts blood flow to our muscles, this ensuring that our blood pressure and fluids remain at an optimal level to work through the possibly harmful situation (Scott, 2020).

Other important parts of the brain to note are the hippocampus, the anterior cingulate cortex, and mirror neurons.

While the amygdala is primarily responsible for emotions, moods, and other functions related to depression and anxiety, the closely attached *hippocampus* is responsible for sending sensory inputs to the amygdala to transmit emotional responses and reactions. The hippocampus functions as a hub for brain network communications, enabling a continuing exchange of information that is correlated with learning and memory (Rubin et al., 2014). It also plays an essential role in the formation of new memories about past experiences and is an important factor in individual and collective group memories, which, as noted in Chapter 4 of this volume, are so potent in the continuance of war (Battaglia et al., 2011).

The *anterior cingulate cortex* has many links to the prefrontal cortex and is associated with detecting errors and thinking about how to resolve conflicts. It is also involved in certain other functions, such as the anticipation of rewards, controlling impulses, and decision-making. Research by Amodio,

Devine, and Harmon-Jones (2008) has outlined its role in the detection and control of race bias.

Mirror neurons are the brain cells that activate when we see someone else doing something, and they try to imitate it. They are an important tool for developing social behavior, as they allow us to understand other people's minds not only through conceptual reasoning but literally by feeling what others are feeling and "living" their emotions (Bernhardt and Singer, 2012). They are an important tool for empathy, which is the ability to understand and share another person's feelings by imagining what it would be like to be in that person's situation. Empathy has been an important element in our survival as a species, enabling us to protect others in our group. Without empathy, it is hard to function as a member of a group; for example, most psychopaths have an empathy deficit, which is why they show a marked lack of concern for their victims. Mirror neurons are more easily activated when we are with people we see as "our" group, but, as we will see in Chapter 4 of this volume, they unfortunately often increase our dislike and fear of people from other groups.

Brain Truth

The advent of machines that can detect our feelings even before we are conscious of them is in itself somewhat humbling, putting to rest the protests of many of us about our supposedly non-prejudiced, rational, and socially inclusive nature. These new machines are able in many cases to tell what our instincts and emotions are more accurately and faster than we ourselves usually can. They are (generally) very honest brokers in assessing the realities of our everyday emotions that for the most part are harmless and go unnoticed—until a challenging context of conflict arises in which they become a huge problem for us, our communities, and our nations.

Functional Magnetic Resonance Imaging

The most important method for testing brain response so far has been fMRI, which measures brain activity by detecting the changes in blood oxygenation and flow that occur in response to neural activity. It can produce maps showing which parts of the brain are involved in a particular mental process and enables scientists to identify which emotion a person is experiencing based on brain activity. It has thus given researchers the first reliable process by which to analyze human emotions. It can identify emotional responses to individuals and other groups that are different to us; many of these responses are largely unknown to us, occurring as they do at an unconscious level. fMRI thus provides unparalleled access to the patterns of brain activity underlying human thinking and behaving in situations of possible tension, confrontation, and conflict.

Electroencephalography

The EEG is a test used to measure brain waves related to electrical activity of the brain. Its successor is quantitative EEG, which can apply more sophisticated mathematical and statistical analysis to these brain waves. Not only can a quantitative EEG track and record brainwave patterns; it can also record an individual's brain activity milliseconds before participants report their intention to act on something (Soon et al., 2008; Verbaarschot et al., 2016). This finding has led to the controversial conclusion that our brain can read our prejudices faster than we can and that it often makes decisions for us even before our own conscious awareness of making them.

Facial Electromyography

Facial electromyography is a technique that measures muscle activity by detecting and amplifying the tiny electrical impulses that are generated by muscle in the face (Kassam et al., 2013). It is a useful tool for measuring and tracking positive and negative emotional reactions to a stimulus as they occur.

The major advantage of the previously discussed techniques is that they can all be used to bypass individuals' own judgments—which are often frighteningly faulty—about their emotions, ideas, and the choices they make. They can circumvent the limitations of traditional methods of self-report, including response biases associated with self-presentational and social desirability concerns (van Hiel, Onraet, and De Pauw, 2010; Jost et al., 2014). They can thus provide us with much more accurate assessments of emotions on many topics of relevance to peacebuilders—for example, prejudice, leadership choices, group responses, and individual and group tendencies toward uncertainty, openness, or closed-mindedness, many of which will be dealt with in later chapters of this book.

It should be noted that all of the previous techniques have their critics. Some researchers assert that determining social/political tendencies from fMRI data are overreaching its capacity and that fMRI machines, one of the most commonly used techniques, are far from ideal for answering questions about the timing and sequence of processing stages (Theodoridis and Nelson, 2012). All neuroimaging techniques are indeed highly susceptible to errors emanating from motions and movements of the body. In addition, the studies are expensive to conduct, so subject pools are frequently small, yielding statistically underpowered and difficult-to-replicate results. Furthermore, the temporal and/or spatial resolution of many techniques is limited. Tasks are often not precisely localized in the brain, and multiple regions may be activated simultaneously, so it is sometimes not easy to attribute specific behaviors to a given brain region or, for that matter, the specific function being activated (Saad and Greengross, 2014). Despite these limitations, these neuroimaging techniques have a proven record for predicting behavior and developing detailed models of human brain organization and function and also for backing up many social psychology theories that appear to have stood the test of time.

The fact that there are now fMRI scanners that can test, describe, and predict with some accuracy how we will think and feel about an issue or an outgroup should give us pause to see how we can use this knowledge to make our peacebuilding work more effective.

Hormonal Truths

Hormonal studies and hormonal testing can also provide fairly accurate assessments of some of the individual and group attitudes and behaviors that are relevant to our work. We now have abundant research that has increased our understanding of how our body chemistry works. One of the relevant systems is the neurochemistry of the brain. The other, which predominates in the rest of the body, is called the endocrine system: glands that produce hormones that are the body's messengers, carrying information and instructions from one set of cells to another. There are over one hundred chemicals at work in the endocrine system that help prepare our bodies for whatever they physically or psychologically need to address any task. These chemical messengers control and affect our emotions.

Many of these hormones, such as cortisol, dopamine, estrogen, melatonin, oxytocin, progesterone, serotonin, testosterone, and vasopressin can influence socially and politically relevant interactions related to attention, communication, feelings, learning, memory, and recognition (Murray, 2017, p. 256). Hormonal studies can now provide us with more accurate assessments of how our hormones relate to individual and group attitudes and relevant behaviors when we are in a context of conflict. These assessments can help us to better understand our responses to messages of fear, our reaction to those we see as "others," and how we are likely to vote (see Chapter 4 of this volume).

The most important hormones relevant to our peacebuilding work are *dopamine*, which is the major transmitter involved in the brain's pleasure pathways (Sharot et al., 2009), and *serotonin*, which appears to be able to stabilize the relationships between the individual and other members of their social group (Koski et al., 2015). Low levels of serotonin are linked to high levels of aggression in men (Duke et al., 2013). The role of *testosterone* is also important, given that most active actors in situations of conflict and war are men. In addition there is *oxytocin*, which is important for positive emotions relating to social bonding and group and intergroup dynamics, as will be noted further in Chapter 3 of this volume.

Genetic Truths

A *gene* is a segment of the molecule that carries most of the instructions used in the development and functioning of the body. DNA (deoxyribonucleic acid) is *a nucleic acid* that determines all the characteristics of a living thing. While a gene is a portion of DNA that determines a certain trait, an *allele* is a specific form of a gene. While genes are responsible for the expression of traits in a person, alleles are responsible for the variations in which a given trait can be expressed. Gene variations appear to strongly influence the way in which we perceive the world, the way we behave, our approach to others, our fear levels, our mental health, and even, eventually, our beliefs and our politics.

Variations in the initial genetic development of our brains are evident as soon as we are born. Several twin studies have linked fear, ethnocentrism, and out-group attitudes with genetic influences on pathogen avoidance and phobias, both of which characteristics affect our perspective on those we see as strangers (Navarrete and Fessler, 2006). Twins were also assessed for social and political attitudes; most of the correlation between social fear and immigration attitudes appeared to be due to a common genetic factor (Orey and Park, 2012). Self-reported racial bias among a sample of European American participants suggested that the short-allele gene variant of 5-HTTLPR predicted greater levels of implicit racial biases (Navarrete and Fessler, 2006). Under stress, 5-HTTLPR is associated with post-traumatic stress disorder and with antisocial behavior (K. Walsh et al., 2014). Research on twin studies has also shown broad gene heritability, which appears to contribute to prosocial behaviors (Rushton, 2004) and to self-reported measures of altruism, cooperativeness, trust, and nurturance (Dawes et al., 2012; Hur and Rushton, 2007; Knafo-Noam et al., 2015; Reuter et al., 2011).

Thus, twin studies very firmly bear out the contention that an individual's social values and beliefs, although not political party affiliations, are to a certain extent genetically related (see Chapters 3 and 4 of this volume). It seems that our genes do not directly affect specific attitudes, but rather genetic tendencies influence how people deal with their emotions toward strangers and out-groups (Hatemi and McDermott, 2012).

Epigenetics

Genes are, of course, not the total determinant of our lives. It appears that after we are born the expression of our genes can be somewhat shaped by our social contexts, although how much such expression is shaped is still a matter of debate (Holmes, 2018; Zhang and Meaney, 2010). The science that looks at the effects of the environment on genes is called *epigenetics* (Duncan, Gluckman, and Dearden, 2014). It is about the mechanism of gene control that can promote or repress the expression of genes without altering their genome's sequence (Feinberg, 2008). Epigenetics looks at the modification of gene expression rather than alteration of the actual DNA genetic code itself. Studies have demonstrated both direct and indirect epigenetic modification as a result of experiences, thus suggesting that genes are not a fixed and unconscious determinant of our biological condition but are responsive to the environment in which we live. The science suggests that in new environments, predisposed genes can experience selection pressures that move some individuals' genes in different *phylogenic* or evolutionary directions than their less flexible peers (Ryan, Hayes, and Craig, 2019). Studies have also begun to exhibit how experience and exposure can cause structural and functional changes in the brain's architecture, thus highlighting its plasticity and capacity for adaptation (Consorti et al., 2019).

It seems that individuals who display a capacity for modifying their behavior as a result of environmental input may be better able to adapt to novel environments than less plastic individuals (Bjorklund, 2006; Mameli, 2004). Also, certain environments may trigger entirely different cognitive or emotive processes or be so powerful that they elicit a common response in humans that leaves little room, at least temporarily, for genetic predispositions. A study of survivors who were highly impacted by the 9/11 attack on the New York World Trade Center found that three times as many reported becoming "more conservative" than "more liberal" in the eighteen months following the strikes (Bonanno and Jost, 2016). A series of studies that focused on gene–environment interplay discovered that where individuals have lost their job, suffered financial loss, or divorced, their support for unions, immigration, capitalism, socialism, and federal housing decreased to almost zero (Hatemi, 2013).

Another field that is looking at the brain in the context of understanding the interplay between the expression of our genes and society is known as *embodied cognitive science*. In this view, both cognitive and emotional processes can be understood only if we look at the whole person in their specific social and cultural environment. This includes prenatal hormones, childhood events, family social and economic conditions, lifetime diet, lifetime environment, and emotional bonding, all of which control the degree to which genes operate and are expressed through behavior (Mateos-Aparicio and Rodríguez-Moreno, 2019). Both epigenetics and embodied cognitive sciences—between which there is considerable overlap—positively suggest that we can create environments that can diminish our predispositions to, for example, being naturally suspicious and fearful of others.

The Brain as a "Confederation of Systems"

The result of the effects of genetic and environmental variants is what Mooney (2012) has described as a "confederation of systems" within the brain, each of different evolutionary age and particular purposes. Alongside the physical adaptions resulting from evolution, we show specialized psychological adaptations that have become ingrained over the course of evolution and have developed to solve problems posed by our environment. We therefore have an older brain designed to respond automatically to danger and to a pressure to "fight or flight," which has been somewhat superseded by a newer brain, designed to make us take cognizant thought of the challenges we face but not always succeeding (Mobbs et al., 2015; also see Chapter 2 of this volume).

The problem for peacebuilders is that if the amygdala becomes the main processor within the brain, people become increasingly vulnerable to manipulation through their emotional responses. Without the capacity to balance their amygdala, fears, and subsequent anger, people become less available to listening to the reasoning of the prefrontal cortex (Banks et al., 2007).

Conclusion

As previously noted, our genes, the architecture of our brain, and our hormonal levels can all affect the reasons and the ways by which we pursue our group and social lives and conflicts. As we have seen, and as will be further developed in the coming chapters, we come into the world with already formed brain and body wiring and chemistry that significantly determines many of our behaviors, beliefs, emotions, relationships, and leadership choices. Those of us who are parents know how variably our differing children will face the world and its challenges; for parents, the "blank slate" hypothesis, which argued that babies were *blank slates* and only had to be taught how to think and behave, has been well and truly discarded (Pinker, 2002). While it is true that our inherited predispositions can be modified by the family and community into which we were born and then, for most of us, can be further modified by our experiences beyond our immediate communities, we know that effecting such personality change can be difficult. It has been likened to turning a supertanker ship (i.e., it can be done, but it can take considerable time and effort). In addition, given the bonuses and pressures of group membership on those who belong to groups, changing group attitudes and behaviors, especially in situations of tension and war, can seem to be a monumental task.

However, the first step in being successful in effecting change is to work with reality—the way people are and not the way we would like them to be or hope they would be. The fact is that almost everyone and every group (excluding perhaps those who are psychopaths) has the capacity within them to turn from hate to cooperation with others, to work together to solve seemingly intractable conflicts, and to choose creative ways to live together as relatively peaceful human beings—or at least human beings who can solve our conflicts through politics, law, and dialogue processes rather than through violence. The fact that there are now well-understood factors tending toward increasing or decreasing such possibilities and fMRI scanners and genetic and hormonal tests that can honestly test, describe, and predict how we will think and feel about an issue or an out-group must give us pause for our peacebuilding work. Ignoring such individual and group predispositions is blind foolishness on our part and will inevitably lead to peacebuilding work that is less effective and less sustainable.

2

The Amygdala Hijack

In our heads we have a rational charioteer who has to rein in an
unruly horse that barely yields to horsewhip and goad combined.

—Plato

Introduction

Between August 6 and 11, 2011, thousands of people rioted across the city
of London. This resulted in the deaths of five people. The disturbances
followed from the police shooting dead a twenty-nine-year old man named
Mark Duggan on August 4. Reports were unclear about why the victim had
been shot, and many people decided to take their anger and frustrations
out on the city. The riots that followed were arguably the worst bout of civil
unrest in a generation. Rioters smashed windows, looted store merchan-
dise, and rampaged the streets, turning over cars and setting them on fire.
Losses in London were indicated to be in the region of £100m (Lock, 2011).
By August 10, more than three thousand arrests had been made, with more
than one thousand people issued with criminal charges for various offences
related to the riots ("England's Week of Riots," 2011). The fact that most of
those caught up in the UK rioting were middle-class teenagers was a surprise
to many. Among those in the dock accused of rioting were "a millionaire's
grammar school daughter, a ballet student, an organic chef, a law student, a
university graduate, a musician and an opera steward" ("The Middle Class
'Rioters' Revealed," 2011).

One of the lawyers subsequently representing the rioters stressed the previously exemplary nature of his clients' characters, telling the court: "I was
taken by surprise. Talking to them and recently talking to their families, they
come across as perfectly ordinary, reasonable, dare I say it civilised young
women" (L. Davies, 2011).

Many of those who took part described a sense of euphoria during the
looting. One young woman said, "It was just everyone was smiling. It was

Our Brains at War. Mari Fitzduff, Oxford University Press (2021). © Oxford University Press.
DOI: 10.1093/oso/9780197512654.003.0003

literally a festival with no food, no dancing, no music but a free shopping trip for everyone." Another said, "After it all kicked off and everyone was doing it, you just joined in and it felt fine. It just felt natural, like you were just naturally shopping." But after the event she handed herself in to the police. Asked what she thought about her actions afterwards, she said "I'm ashamed. To think that I went that low to go steal in these shops when they're, like, basically that's their business, that's how they're providing for their families, and we've basically ruined that and they've got to start from scratch" ("Reading the Riots," 2011, pp. 28–29).

It is not uncommon that in the wake of riots that people who have participated wonder at themselves and at the damage they may have committed. They are confused because they did not believe that such behavior was part of their "real" character. In the case of the London riots, there was indeed no evidence that any of those involved in the rioting were normally violent characters or mentally unstable. It appears that the situation had shocked or seduced them into behavior that they subsequently felt was unnatural to them. But was it? Apparently, or so research now tells us, the answer is no—it was not unnatural. All of us, no matter our class or creed, can be easily caught up emotionally in the power of a situation. Afterwards we might well ask ourselves, "Who exactly is in charge of our behavior?" "Us," we will say, of course—but which "us"?

In every person and, by extension, every group, our "emotional" and "reasoning" minds coexist uneasily. Our human existence throughout history was often dependent not on rationality but on instincts and emotions. An oncoming tiger or a warring neighbor with bow and arrow does not give much time for reflection. Our survival depended on our emotional instinct as to how to respond, and such instincts usually kick in before the more rational part of our mind has time to draw breath. Despite such frequent reminders as temper losses, road rage, overeating, or falling in love, we often find it hard to accept this. However, being instinctual is often unconscious, and our default particularly when we are together as part of a group—at football matches, social and political rallies, riots, wars, etc. Most of us fail to understand how precarious the conscious/rational side of our brains is, until we find ourselves in a context that unleashes the forces of our amygdala. In situations of conflict and violence, and often preceding such, where our families, communities, and people feel under stress, fear and group processes often overtake our emotions. These emotions can be extremely hard to control, particularly at group level and in situations where feelings of threat are to the fore—which is the case in most violent and conflicted situations.

This challenge has been well captured by Haidt in his analogy of the elephant and the rider, where our emotional side is the elephant, and our rational, reasonable side is the rider (Haidt, 2006). The rider is perched atop the elephant and seems to be the leader, but control is precarious because the rider is so small and so new relative to the much older elephant. Any time the elephant and the rider disagree about which direction to go, the amygdala/elephant part of our brain is likely to win, unless we are able to bring the prefrontal cortex/reasoning part of our brain strongly to bear on our decisions. As noted in Chapter 1 of this volume, our amygdala (the part of the brain that processes our automatic/intuitive emotional impulses) and prefrontal cortex (which deals with our conscious/reasoned/logical responses to a situation) both struggle to gain our attention and modify our behavior.

Electroencephalogram and hormonal testing reveal clearly that we are more at the mercy of our amygdalate tendencies, particularly in times of tension, when we mostly take our cues from what we feel rather than what we think (DeLaRosa et al., 2014; Mooney, 2012a). In situations of possible danger, our amygdala will usually gain traction first.

We are particularly at the mercy of our emotions when we meet people who are obviously different to us (see Chapter 3 of this volume). We often decide what we think of people with just a glance, judging them instantly. "We decide very quickly whether a person possesses many of the traits we feel are important, such as likeability and competence, even though we have not exchanged a single word with them. It appears that we are hard-wired to draw these inferences in a fast, unreflective way" (Boutin, 2006).

"We imagine trust to be a rather sophisticated response, but our observations indicate that trust might be a case of a high-level judgment being made by a low-level brain structure. Perhaps the signal bypasses the cortex altogether" (Willis and Todorov, 2006). Thus it appears that our initial or group emotions are often governed by biological influences, particularly in situations of strangeness or tension, which ensure that our emotions take control and run an automatic response program—what is called an "emotional hijack."

Emotional Hijack

An emotional hijack is what appears to have happened to many of the London rioters. It refers to a situation in which the amygdala—the part of the brain that serves as our emotional processor—hijacks or bypasses our normal reasoning process to respond intuitively to a situation, sometimes termed a "fight or flight" response to possible imminent danger (Cannon, 1915, p. 211). There is a logic to such hijacking when one is being chased by a tiger or in a situation where our families, communities or nations feel threatened. When a danger presents itself, we need simply and urgently to act in whatever way best increases our chance of survival. When such an emotional hijack happens

> we notice immediate changes like an increased heart rate or sweaty palms. Our breathing becomes more shallow and rapid as we take in more oxygen, preparing to bolt if we have to. . . . The active amygdala also immediately shuts down the neural pathway to our prefrontal cortex so we can become disoriented in a heated conversation. Complex decision-making disappears, as does our access to multiple perspectives. (Hamilton, 2015)

This tension between intuitive/emotive thinking and cognitive reasoning has been highlighted by Kahneman (2011), who termed it "fast versus slow thinking." According to Kahneman, our minds operate essentially from two systems: System 1, which operates automatically, quickly, and instinctually and is not usually under our control, and System 2, which is where our ideas and responses are generated consciously by the self. System 2 usually includes a consideration of future perspectives, as well as memories that are relevant to the situation to respond or take decisions about actions. Interestingly, it seems that these two systems also correlate with the kinds of moral judgments that people ultimately make about others—that is, we feel the emotion and then seek logical reasons to uphold our moral thinking (Greene, 2011, pp. 125–128; Lewis et al., 2012).

We usually have no choice over such instinctual feelings. Our feelings are generally dictated to us not only by our brain structures but also by our hormones such as adrenaline, norepinephrine, and cortisol, which inform our responses to fear messages. Many of our initial reactions to such negative stimuli and information are automatically set in motion prior to (and often in the absence of) conscious thought (Jung et al., 2014). It is only after a mindful awareness of the stimulus, approximately half a second from the original exposure, that a person can begin self-regulation to try to overcome such scripted patterns of behavior (Lack and Bogacz, 2012, http://lawtech. ch/wp-content/uploads/2016/03/J.-Lack-F.-Bogacz-The-Neurobiology-of-Conflict-2012-Cardozo-JCR.pdf).

It does appear that such strong emotions can subsequently be tempered by emotional self-regulation, normally implemented by a neural circuit comprising various prefrontal regions and subcortical limbic structures (Beauregard, Lévesque, and Bourgouin, 2001). Thus it appears that humans do have the capacity to influence the electrochemical dynamics of their brains by voluntarily changing the nature of the processes of reflection. In other words, while we are often not responsible for what we feel, we can be responsible for how we react to our feelings.

However, another problem to such reflection by the cortex is that in normal life we are frequently distracted and running on autopilot in much of our decision-making. Our minds are often dependent on a range of hardwired biases and heuristics that distort our reality and our decisions (Kahneman, 2011). And, given that our emotions precede, and often trump, our rational conscious thoughts, these feelings can quickly determine our behavior, which we will then often use our belated reasoning capacity to justify. Thus when we argue, supposedly with the assistance of our cortex, our arguments are often driven by emotions and memories we can hardly recollect.

Brains Differ

It is important to note that while the previously noted tension between our emotional and reasoning sides is present in all humans, their varying pressures can differ widely from person to person. Many of these differences are determined by our genetic inheritances (Mendez, 2017). Functional magnetic resonance imaging scans have shown that these differences in biology influence differences in attitudes and beliefs. In challenging situations, some people show an increased volume of activity in the amygdala, while others show an increased grey matter volume in the cortex. Studies have shown that these genetic differences can be observed from birth. Even as babies, those with a naturally larger amygdala response respond much more quickly to sudden noises and threatening visual images, while others can tolerate fear and uncertainty more easily. To trust and cooperate primarily with members of one's own group is the easier choice for those whose amygdala responses are generally more fearful and for whom trusting people from other groups is harder. "Fearful people who dislike uncertainty and who are wary of strangers, and of things that they do not understand, are more likely to be supportive of policies that give them a sense of security" (Hatemi et al., 2013).

Such people, often called conservatives or traditionalists, tend to have a greater need for order, structure, and certainty in their lives; resist change more often; and are less open to risk-taking. They report greater physiological levels of disgust when faced with bugs or blood and in relation to such issues as gay marriage and abortion. They often highly value "purity" and order and are known to devote high levels of attention to norm violations. Such attitudes can be very conducive to establishing and reinforcing a them-and-us conflict. It has been suggested that the Taliban originally emerged out of the disgust felt by former pious mujahedeen living in Pakistan at the lives of their fellow citizens whom they saw as socially and morally corrupt and impure. Thus was born the commitment of the Taliban, and subsequently ISIS/Islamic State, to establishing a "pure" Islamic state, with no compromises, through the use of sharia law. Individuals with greater physiological responses are also more likely to take conservative positions such as supporting capital punishment and high defense spending, support for the Iraq War, and patriotism (Oxley et al., 2008). Thus they also tend to be more supportive of anti-immigration and pro-segregation policies (Hatemi et al., 2013; also see Chapter 4 of this volume).

On the other hand there are, in all societies, a seemingly different type of people, generally called liberals, who differ on a continuum from conservatives in terms of their physiological responses to stimuli, brain function, and even static brain anatomy (Taber and Young, 2013, p. 541). When faced with a conflict they are more likely than conservatives to be more flexible and to alter their habitual response when cues indicate it is necessary (Amodio et al., 2007).

Researchers have identified a gene variant called DRD4-7R, which affects the neurotransmitter called dopamine. Individuals carrying it are more likely to turn out to be more open-minded people and to get special pleasure from variety, novelty, and diversity (Settle et al., 2010).

Thus, it now seems clear that political behaviors and attitudes such as out-group preferences and political trust are not simply the result of socialization but also are part of an individual's genetically informed disposition (Klemmensen et al., 2012). While the predisposition to experience greater fear has a biophysical component, what exactly people will fear, or which groups they will hate, will differ depending on their history, their culture, and their social environment. "Elections are decided in the marketplace of emotions, a marketplace filled with values, images, analogies, moral sentiments, and moving oratory, in which logic plays only a supporting role" (Westen, 2008).

Group Emotions

It is important to note that individuals' emotions can easily spread to others. Evidence from neuroscience suggests that the pattern of neuronal firing in the brain of a given individual can mirror that of another individual that they are observing or with whom they are interacting (Iacoboni, 2009). Thus people who are simply observing or in the presence of another individual who is performing an activity or experiencing a certain emotion can become infected with that emotion through a process called "emotional contagion"—that is, the process by which emotions are transferred automatically and unconsciously between individuals to form a group pattern that can help to explain group demonstrations, riots, and genocides (Peterson et al., 2015; Murray, 2017; Reina, Peterson, and Waldman, 2015). The effect of such "emotional contagion" is often obvious in those attending political or group rallies, where the prevailing emotional atmosphere is often one of excitement, bonding, and finding enemies. Faces of participants at a Donald Trump rally are an interesting example of such emotions.

Such emotional contagion can be assisted not only from current situations but also through memories that in many cases have been generated, fostered, and evoked by many decades of conflict. Volkan (2001) talks about collective memories and narrative of victimhood and of how they can be transmitted emotionally from one generation to the next in what calls a "chosen trauma"—that is, the mental representation of an event that has caused a large group to "face drastic losses, feel helpless and victimized by another group, and share a humiliating injury" (Volkan, 1998, p. 4). Such memories can easily be hooked into group contagion, can easily be evoked by leaders, and can become the emotional underpinning for the motivation of groups, often assisted by such processes as battle reminiscences, storytelling, and nationalist music and symbols.

Why Differing Brains?

Why do some people have brains that are more naturally fearful than others? There is speculation in the literature that in evolutionary terms it may have proved useful to have such varied types of individuals in a society to ensure the best survival responses to different sets of societal and group challenges. A society that was made up of people completely of one disposition, either conservatives or liberals, is unlikely to survive. People who have no fear of strangers and whose amygdalae have been completely destroyed appear to feel that everyone is "my kind" and feel no threats from out-groups (McCloskey, 2015). A lack of such feelings would obviously, throughout history, leave them open to possible manipulation, abuse, and killing, which would make the group's survival less likely. On the other hand, society needs people who are of a more conservative disposition and who can continue processes and institutions that seemed to have worked throughout their history and which they deem should not be put easily aside. It is notable that people who are more conservative have been the majority norm throughout history, and it has been suggested that that the more recent growth in liberalism may be viewed as an evolutionary luxury that is increasingly afforded only by the fact that many societies are becoming less deadly today (Doolittle, 2016). The slow growth in liberalism in the Unites States and many other democratic countries would seem to validate this idea.

The Thrills of Combat

For many participants in the London riots mentioned at the beginning of this chapter, such riots will have been exciting, permitting them to give in to emotions normally kept under control. As one reporter covering the riots said,

> for many of those who took part in the riots, it will have been one of the great experiences of their lives. For riots, even more than strikes, provide people who have often lived desolate, atomised, boring lives with an experience of solidarity, of collective power, of being able to affect the course of society at large instead of merely being on the receiving end. (Harman, 1981)

Thus it is important for people to understand that being involved in a riot, or being militarily involved in a war, including the very act of killing, attempting to kill, or being killed, can provide a "high" of meaning in the lives of many perpetrators. My own PhD focus was on paramilitaries and others in Northern Ireland who had renounced violence as a way to change society (Fitzduff, 1989). Almost all the paramilitaries who were interviewed said (somewhat shamefacedly) that they had never felt more "alive" than while out with their "active service units," or their "killing missions" as others might call such activities. While they had now eschewed violence, they missed being part of an active group that had given their lives both thrills and meaning.

Such positive feelings are not unusual on the part of veterans of both legal and illegal ilk. MacNair (2006), who researched the reactions of US veterans to killing, echoes this: "It does appear from much clinical observation that killing can at the same time be traumatic in its long-term effects on the mind and yet still have the immediate effect of a sensation of exhilaration, a sense of the thrill of the kill, a combat high" (p. 198). In fact, some of the men (they are mostly men—see Chapter 7 of this volume) can actually become addicted to such killing highs. Silva et al. (2001) refers to it as an "action-addiction" syndrome on the part of many veterans in what they call "a behavioral pattern involving aggression where the affected individual seeks to re-experience thoughts, feelings and actions related to previous combat experiences" (p. 313). It has even been suggested that the addiction could be biochemical in nature, as war often gives men a high of exhilaration and power. Many of these apparently addicted veterans "openly regard civilian life with contempt and think of it as being mundane and inconsequential" (Glover, 1985, p. 17).

Others too can become addicted. Chris Hedges, a veteran journalist of many wars, says that "there is a part of me that remains nostalgic for war's simplicity and high. . . . The enduring attraction of war is this: Even with its destruction and carnage it gives us what we all long for in life. It gives us purpose, meaning, a reason for living" (Hedges, 2002, p. 3). Unless peacebuilders realize this attraction for war on the part of many who become legal or illegal soldiers (see Chapter 5 of this volume), we will fail in our peacebuilding strategies and our post-war rehabilitation programs. We need to remember that the need for such highs, meaning, and belonging will often continue after the war unless previous militarists find alternative outlets, such as politics, for their needs and skills.

The New Challenge to Our
Cortex: Social Media

There is a new kind of war facing nations today, in which hard weaponry may well play second fiddle to the use of social media by governments and other groups to enhance the moods and emotions of citizens involved in conflicted contexts (see Chapter 8 of this volume). Twitter and Facebook have demonstrated the power of their platforms through manipulating their users' emotions just by changing their news feed and through the process of emotional contagion (Booth, 2014). Such power is unprecedented in the history of humankind and has potentially disastrous consequences in terms of war and peacebuilding.

It seems that social media platform algorithms prioritize posts that contain strong emotions, thus spreading their messages at vast speeds to millions of others (Nicas, 2018). Such platforms often bypass the rational parts of our minds and "speak instead to the emotional, reactive, quick-fix parts of us, that are satisfied by images and clicks that look pleasing, that feed our egos, and that make us think we are heroic" (Golumbia, 2018). The advent of social media and its "race to the brainstem" ("Optimizing for Engagement," 2019) makes emotional persuasion easier and complex thinking more difficult. This is particularly true when there are societal tensions, and we become easy prey for purveyors of conflict who wish to emotionally persuade us to support their particular goals or objectives. Thus our human social and neurological tendencies and needs can easily be hijacked by those who seek to use social media to deleteriously affect others. It was through a very sophisticated use of social media that ISIS/Daesh was so successful in recruiting thousands of young men, and some women, to its cause.

Given that emotions—particularly fearful emotions—are contagious, it can be easily seen how a dedicated group of social media savvies can incite a war. In Rwanda, a radio was enough to help start a genocide (Kellow and Steeves, 1998). Wars are already being distorted by social media processes, and such distortions will be an important part of future wars (see Chapter 9 of this volume).

Conclusion

As shown in the studies of Kahneman (2011) and many others, undermining the "rationality myth" is enormously difficult since most of us like to perceive ourselves as rational creatures. The possibility that instinct and feelings determine some of the most important decisions we make in our lives is probably hard for many readers to digest. However, by understanding the human predisposition toward emotions as opposed to rationality we just may be able to strategize our work more effectively. At the very least we may save our breath by not reasoning too long with those whose positions are born from emotions like fear. It appears that in the main, we would be better understanding the feelings behind their arguments rather than the facts, and such understanding may suggest different approaches that may be more productive.

Like many others in our peacebuilding field, I have filing cabinets full of "solutions" to our own and other conflicts around the world. I have seen most of the imaginative maps for the conflicts in Israel/Palestine, North/South Sudan, the former Yugoslavia, Cameroon, Northern Ireland, etc., showing the possibilities for ending these conflicts. However, I have long ago learned that the problem is not that there are not "solutions" to these conflicts—there usually are many—but that the prior and often harder task is getting people emotionally as well as rationally engaged in approaching the filing cabinet and its full quota of solutions together.

In basing our work mostly on rational/logical thinking, we often fail to understand how little sway such thinking has on leaders. Peace agreements often fall apart because, although the cognitive skills of those involved have crafted clever political and social compromises, when leaders return to their land or their people, the emotions necessary for the agreement to be sustainable are lacking. Thus, crises that arise in the implementation of such agreements often return leaders and their constituencies to the emotions that have helped to kindle and sustain the violence in the first place.

3

Us and Others

Biologically humans have evolved for cooperation—but only with some people.

—Greene (2011)

Introduction

Between 1941 and 1945, Ustaše militias and death squads burned villages and killed thousands of civilian Serbs living in the Croatian countryside. Men, women, and children were hacked to death, thrown alive into pits and down ravines, or set on fire in churches. People in Serbian villages near Srebrenica and Ozren were entirely massacred while children were found impaled on stakes in villages between the towns of Vlasenica and Kladanj (Yeomans, 2005). The Ustaše cruelty and sadism shocked even Nazi commanders. A Gestapo report to Reichsführer SS Heinrich Himmler, dated February 17, 1942, said,

> The Ustaše committed their deeds in a bestial manner not only against males of conscript age, but especially against helpless old people, women and children. The number of the Orthodox that the Croats have massacred and sadistically tortured to death is about three hundred thousand. (Goñi, 2002, p. 202)

Many of those killed by the Croats had previously been their neighbors and friends. So how had this happened? Unfortunately, it is likely that the killers were assisted in their finding of old and new enemies by the nature of their human genes, the functioning of their brains, and the turbulence of their hormones. These are factors that were useful to every nation or group in history when they set out to conduct a war against a group defined as an "enemy."

Our Brains at War. Mari Fitzduff, Oxford University Press (2021). © Oxford University Press.
DOI: 10.1093/oso/9780197512654.003.0004

Our Human Bias

Evolutionary social psychology, which is a combination of social and evolutionary psychology, as well as evolutionary biology (Schaller, Simpson, and Kenrick, 2014) is based on the Darwinian assumption that our personal and social psychology is the product of evolution through natural selection. It suggests that in the same way that the body adapted to evolutionary needs, so did the mind, to solve the problems posed by our changing social and environmental contexts. The idea that our minds have been honed by evolution may be problematic to some, but if we accept that the brain is part of the body, it is logically consistent to argue that the human brain has been shaped by our environment.

Given what we are learning through the new biosciences, it appears that that our human brains, as well as having a tendency to respond instinctively to often unnoticed emotions, as noted in Chapter 2 of this volume, have developed a need for group bonding, which provides us with many of the benefits that we crave as human beings (e.g., security, meaning, and belonging). However, to define our in-group we need to find an out-group: this categorization of out-groups into enemies or friends, part of our group or not part of our group, is a universal trait that takes place in all communities, societies, and nations. While religion and cultural and social ideologies often bind a group together, they are not necessary to the development of group boundaries—almost any categorization will do. Out-group identification can be based on race, class, gender and gender orientation, uniforms, language, religion, culture, ethnicity, geographic location, etc. Even the apparently smallest of social, historical, or theological differences, such as those between Sunni or Shia Muslims, can and do provide a framework for violent social conflict in many parts of the world. One's pronunciation of a particular word can in many places be enough of a marker to kill or be killed; for example, in biblical times, the Gileadites would test the Ephraimites to pronounce a word correctly as the only way to tell their enemy from their friend (Judges 12:6).[1]

Our framing of an out-group will of course differ and change from context to context; for example, people from Ireland and Italy were not considered "white" by most nineteenth-century Americans, and it took a US court to decide in 1909 that Armenians were part of the "white" race. In many countries

---

[1] https://biblehub.com/judges/12-6.htm

people whose gender orientation is deemed not to be of a "normal" female/male nature can still be imprisoned and killed.

Ample evidence of this tendency of group need has been provided time and again in experiments carried out by social psychologists. The Stanford Prison experiment by Zimbardo and his colleagues (Zimbardo et al., 1973) was set up to test just how we as humans will respond to contexts in which our group membership is ethically tested. In the study, volunteers were assigned to be either "guards" or "prisoners" in a mock prison. The subjects quickly embraced their assigned roles, with many "guards" becoming sadistic and psychologically abusive toward the "prisoners," while many "prisoners" passively accepted such abuse and even, at the request of the role-playing "officers," actively harassed their fellow "prisoners" who tried to stop it. The experiment was abandoned after six days as the organizers became concerned for the safety of the "normal" volunteers, whose personalities appeared in most cases to have taken a turn for the worse in the mock prison context. The experiment seemed to confirm that the most normal of us human beings can be turned into vicious, cruel people in certain contexts.

How easy it is to divide us from each other was also evidenced by Muzafer Sherif and colleagues in the Robber's Cave experiment, in which boys were randomly split into two groups who were given competing goals (Sherif et al., 1961). This process alone quickly generated hostilities between the groups, which became enemies within hours of being randomly separated, and soon began to be openly hostile to each other. It appears that a greater awareness of almost any group membership brings not only an increased preference for all things that are particular to one's group but also the easy scapegoating of both non-conforming in-group members and of members of other groups.

Why is this? It seems that most individuals locate themselves and others into social categories and that the simple act of categorizing individuals into groups is sufficient for the emergence of an "us" and "them" division. This theory became known as social identity theory (Tajfel, 1978). People will, of course, often have more than one identity that is important to them, and these identifications may overlap. However, the salience and importance of one or other membership will vary considerably, depending on the context. In times of conflict, particular identities usually become more simplistic and more fundamental to the individual's concept of their self, and it becomes harder for people to see their group identity as negotiable. This, in conjunction with real or perceived grievances, fosters large-scale hostility, whereby even neighbors who have been closely associated with one another through friendship or marriage become deep enemies. According to Waller (2006, p. 90), experiments like Zimbardo's point to the disturbing fact that "as collectives, we engage in acts of extraordinary evil, with apparent moral calm and intensity of supposed purpose, which could only be described as insane were they committed by an individual." He also notes that moral constraints are less powerful in groups than in individuals and that this can make it easier for the members to group people with a moral authority that can give individuals sufficient justification to perpetrate harm or "extraordinary evil" upon them.

Why the Importance of Group Membership?

Why have we inherited brains that are so inherently sensitive to out-group affiliation? For most of the millions of years that our species has been developing, we have lived and apparently thrived through our membership of smallish groups, and thus evolution appears to have inculcated within us a deep need to belong to, and relate to, such groups. It also seems that we always seek an out-group, perhaps because in-group favoritism, in combination with out-group hostility, seems to have emerged as a highly successful survival strategy (Choi and Bowles, 2007). A collective belief framework also appears to help a strategy of survival. It is usually our geographic location, our social context, and our relationships with our families and our communities and nations that will determine in the first instance what we believe, how we normally behave, and who we hate. We mostly draw on our own community for a pattern of beliefs such as religion, culture, or nationalism that have seemingly worked well for our group in the past and contributed to our group survival. These socially influenced ways of thinking and behaving usually become second nature to us. Without even thinking or choosing, we take our beliefs and our ways of working as an understanding of right and natural behavior, not least because for us to move significantly outside of our community norms and beliefs involves exclusion and possible danger. Given the importance of group belonging, people usually moderate their beliefs so as to conform to the groups to which they belong, or want to belong, and within which membership implies relative safety. It thus appears that most religions and many ideological beliefs are geographic beliefs rather than proven "true" beliefs.

Belonging to a group provides an important positive function for human beings:

> It fulfils deep needs and provides satisfactions inherent in connection with others. It provides a feeling of security. It is essential in defining the self as a member of a family, a profession, a religious group, voluntary associations, and a nation. Individual identity is defined and the self gains value and significance through identification with groups and the connection to others that membership provides. (Staub, 1989, p. 252)

Staub points to research that shows that such group support—whether it is a group of fellow concentration camp victims or companions working for a shared cause—contributes positively to survival even under the worst of conditions. Own group survival, which goes beyond kinship, is critical for humans to cooperate, to build villages and cities, to reproduce and have families, and to defend themselves and their territories against threats to their group. The degree to which people identify with a cultural or ethnic group can serve as a buffer against environmental stresses (Decety et al., 2018). The importance of racial identification to psychological well-being, educational outcomes, and physical health can be particularly adaptive for minorities living in multicultural communities. For instance, African Americans often demonstrate increased racial identification in response to increased perceived racial discrimination. Heightened identification with other racial minority group members can also increase academic performance (C.O. Smith et al., 2009) and decrease risk for cardiovascular disease (Chae et al., 2010). However, such identification can be reflexive and difficult to override (Ito and Urland, 2005), not least because breaking social norms would usually create shame and stigma for the person doing it.

The problem is that when the brain creates an "us" in terms of group membership, it actively needs an out-group against which to define its identity (Appiah, 2018). The need to belong is even stronger when there is tension and violence in societies, when it is frighteningly easy for groups to take sides, often in opposition to each other and at the expense of previously close relationships. It appears that our often latent group biases, such as race or other identity biases, may be a fear "prepared" by evolution because way back in our histories we were aware that contact with different groups could bring danger. Some researchers have suggested that this could be because of the fear of out-group germs: the pathogen stress theory (Thornhill and Fincher, 2014). Its logic suggests that

> throughout human evolutionary history, members of unfamiliar out-groups are likely to have posed significant disease threats. . . . Consistent with theories emphasizing the pernicious dangers potentially posed by out-group pathogens, this bias was strongest if the targets were also a part of a racial out-group. Findings suggest a fundamental link between disease avoidance processes and biases in intergroup cognition. (Makhanova, Miller, and Maner, 2015, p. 18)

Such threats can also be a fear re limited resources of land and food. For example, Rwanda before the genocide in 1994 was one of the most densely populated countries in Africa, and many of the tensions that undelay this conflict were about such land pressures (Takeuchi and Marara, 2009). Thus our often fearful pre-judgments can be seen as a survival mechanisms that predispose us to fear out-groups and the possible threat they pose to our survival and that of our family and communities.

The Advent of Functional Magnetic Resonance Imaging

The relatively recent application of neuroscience to the study of social categorization has provided important insights into the specific processes that underlie intergroup categorization. It appears that our brains are inherently sensitive to group affiliation. This means that neural structures often amplify the prejudice and fear we feel about people who are different from us. In many situations, our bodies are ahead of us in such feelings, and our group memberships affect our neural processes automatically and unconsciously.

It appears that the amygdala, the insula, and the ventral striatum all play substantial roles in partisan bias, racial prejudice, intergroup relations, and individual decisions about attitudes (Tusche et al., 2013; Zamboni et al., 2009). Thus, when we meet people or groups who are different to us, our amygdala rapidly processes social category cues in terms of potential threat or reward, with attendant emotional responses. These processes have important implications for discriminatory behavior (Cunningham et al., 2004).

Several functional magnetic resonance imaging (fMRI) studies of social categorization have demonstrated an "out-group race face" bias in a brain—that is, black and white perceivers exhibited relatively greater amygdala activity when viewing other-race faces than own-race faces (Ronquillo et al., 2007). Responses to out-group members appear to be characterized by reduced activity in the ventromedial prefrontal cortex, a region that is involved in empathy and mentalizing (Amodio, 2014). When we meet people or groups who are different to us, our amygdala rapidly processes social category cues in terms of potential threat or reward, with attendant emotional responses toward those we perceive as others. In addition, activation in the anterior cingulate cortex increases when a person has an automatic negative response to an out-group member (Krill and Platek, 2009). Interestingly, If the dorsolateral prefrontal cortex, which controls our emotional responses, is suppressed through transcranial magnetic stimulation—a changing magnetic field used to cause electric current in a specific area of the brain (Millar, 2012)—a person's expression of bias toward another person or group will be increased (Fecteau et al., 2007). "Thus when confronted with, for example, a black American, white Americans often experience an automatic fear response—one that they are often unaware of and do not necessarily condone" (Bruneau, 2016).

It seems that we have inherited brains that are inherently sensitive to group affiliation and find security and comfort with those who share our identities. Thus, the use of, for example, in-group words compared to out-group words activates a specific network including the ventral medial prefrontal and anterior and dorsal cingulate cortex. These regions correspond to a neural network previously identified as the "personal self"; this network apparently derives much of our self-image from the groups we belong to (Morrison, Decety, and Molenberghs, 2012).

Unfortunately, those of us who are prejudiced toward one group are likely to be prejudiced to most out-groups. Two studies that investigated out-group–to–out-group generalization (i.e., out-group projection; Albarello et al., 2017) looked at whether members of negatively perceived minority out-groups are perceived as prototypical of larger partially inclusive out-groups and whether this tendency is enhanced under intergroup threat. Both tested prejudice against the Roma as being predictive of prejudice against Arabs.

These responses appear to be universal. Many studies done with people of different ethnic backgrounds indicate the widespread nature of our racial or color bias. These include studies that have compared responses between

Hispanic and black and white participants, black participants with white and Japanese participants, Chinese with Korean and white participants, Chinese with Indian and other East Asian ethnic participants (Perera-W.A., 2016), Turkish and German participants, and Arab and Israeli Jews (Brigham et al., 2007). All these studies have come to the same conclusion—that all races notice and respond to physical differences in others. Just how different other people are to us is also important: the greater the difference, the deeper the prejudicial response. Research has shown that brain activity in the amygdala and anterior insula was positively correlated with the objective "blackness" of faces: the "blacker" the other face, the greater was the insula activity (Ronquilla et al., 2007). And, as previously noted, extreme whiteness, such as that of albinos, can also provoke fear and violence.

Not only do we respond to those who are different, but we also respond almost instantaneously—our judgments often take just a fraction of a second (Amodio, 2014). Numerous experiments confirm that the brain differentially processes images within milliseconds based on minimum cues about race or gender. Just one-fifty millisecond exposure to the face of another race activates the amygdala. Our brains form us/them categories at stunning speed but nevertheless set our attitudes in such a way that stereotypes and prejudices can all too easily be established. Such automatic judgment processing helps explain why bias stubbornly persists even if our current beliefs tell us it is wrong.

These results also suggest that of the two systems of thinking suggested by Kahneman (see Chapter 2 of this volume), it is the fast, automatic processing that is involved in racial bias. Negative or positive feelings toward other groups are often instinctual and outside our consciousness, and thus tamping them down requires extra mental effort (Phelps et al., 2000). Unfortunately, because such fear-conditioned responses are expressed primarily in autonomic responses (e.g., increased heart rate), they can be learned very rapidly, often after a single exposure to the stimulus in a threatening context, and such associations may be difficult to extinguish (Schiller et al., 2013).

From an evolutionary perspective, heightened sensitivity to in-group fear expressions serves an important function in coordinating group action in response to danger. A meta-analysis revealed that individuals are better at recognizing and understanding the emotions expressed by their cultural ingroup compared with their cultural out-group (Chiao et al., 2008). There is greater activity in regions of the brain associated with emotion processing when people are asked to identify the emotions of their co-nationals versus those of foreigners (Chiao et al., 2008; Freeman et al., 2009). There may be an "in-group advantage" in such emotion recognition (Mesquita and Leu, 2007). From an evolutionary perspective, heightened sensitivity to in-group fear expressions serves an important function in coordinating group action in response to danger.

Thus, unless we are very used to living in an identity-diverse context, in which case we have often learned to discount initial feelings of fear and bias, we should assume that initially reacting with caution to groups that are seen as "other" to our group is normal and hope that we are increasingly able to elicit the rationality of our prefrontal cortex to guide our future feelings and actions.

Some OF Us Are More Prejudiced Than Others

While all of us are inclined to notice and react to differences in others, it seems that some of us will react more negatively to groups seen as out-groups. In all societies there are those who favor engagement with out-groups and those who see such groups as threats to be to be avoided—as we have seen in Chapter 2 of this volume, some of us are intrinsically more fearful than others.

It appears that basic individual differences in reactivity to threatening or aversive stimuli are predictors of individual differences in racial bias. Research on the influence of the serotonin transporter polymorphism (5-HTTLPR) on implicit and self-reported racial bias among a sample of European American participants suggested that the short-allele variant of 5-HTTLPR predicted greater levels of implicit racial biases but not explicit self-reported racial biases (i.e., the responses were unconscious and not reflected in the self-reporting of such bias).

Such reactivity is particularly evident when people have had no previous contact with members of different social groups such as people who look black or Arab and particularly when allied with their perception of a dangerous social environment. Such reactions provide evidence of a gene–environment model of intergroup bias. In particular they demonstrate the key role of a specific gene, the serotonin transporter polymorphism, in the development of unconscious prejudice, particularly in the face of an environmental threat (Cheon et al., 2014, pp. 1268–1275).

Such higher fear levels can play a significant role in influencing attitudes on issues such as immigration, law and order, and capital punishment, as we will see in Chapter 4 of this volume.

Empathy Neurons

Given the importance and benefits of belonging, it appears that our bodies are set to help us to maintain our membership of a group, particularly if we tend to be of a more fearful disposition. This means that biologically humans may have evolved for useful cooperation—but mainly with those they see as their in-group. This has led some researchers to claim that we are wired for tribalism, which may be a challenge in today's increasingly globalizing world.

Such a suggestion would seem to be plausible when observing the actions of our mirror neurons. These neurons are a small circuit of cells in the premotor cortex and inferior parietal cortex of the brain that are automatically mobilized when we feel our own pain and also when we feel the pain of (some) others (Acharya and Shukla, 2012). They are the part of the neural circuitry that provides our emotional response to the distress or excitement of other people. Before the discovery of mirror neurons, scientists generally believed that it was through the use of our brains and cognitive thought processes that we interpreted and predicted other people's behavior. Now, however, many have come to believe that we understand others not by thinking, but by feeling through the "mirror" neurons in the affective brain circuits. These neurons are linked to our capacity for empathy, the emotion that enables us to better understand other people's intentions and feelings and allows us to see the world from another's point of view. Brain imaging experiments using fMRI have shown that these are active when the person performs an action and also when they see another individual performing an action. The same activation of neurons occurs in an observer to that that is occurring in a person doing an action (e.g., playing a sport—hence the excitement for followers) or expressing a facial emotion (e.g., grimacing; Lack and Bogacz, 2011).

A meta-analysis by researchers has indicated that a core network consisting of bilateral anterior insular cortices and medial/anterior cingulate cortex is associated with empathy, or lack of empathy, for pain, depending on in-group or out-group status (Lamm et al., 2011; Mattan et al., 2018). Thus, when we encounter people from groups we perceive as strangers to us, and in particular those we see as threatening to us in some way, the brain often switches off the empathetic mirror neurons completely and actively resists any emotional connection with the perceived "other" group (Bobula, 2011; Bruneau and Saxe, 2010)· fMRI studies of the neural impulses of interaction and empathy between individuals of different perceived group backgrounds and membership have shown a lower degree or even a complete absence of mirror neural activity when groups are perceived to be different (Bobula, 2011; Xu et al., 2009). The amount of empathy we show another person is thus often decided by our social relationship with that person (Bobula, 2011).

Our ability to empathetically perceive and respond to the affective states of another emerges as early as two years of age (Svetlova, Nichols, and Brownell, 2010). Its existence appears to a universally hard-wired response, although its expression will vary with cultural context. It is interesting to note that the part of the brain that controls empathy appears to be bigger in women, who show enhanced empathetic ability compared to males (Schulte-Rüther et al., 2008).

Our innate tendency toward in-group bias is echoed in sociological studies that have studied high levels of integration or "bonding" social capital—that is, the networks of relationships among people who live and work in a particular society. It appears that the deeper such networks are, the more they seem to reduce a group's capacity to develop "bridging" and cooperation, between differing identity groups (Putnam, 2000). Thus, while "bonding" social capital may involve norms and trust, it can also serve as a lock-in mechanism that isolates people and groups from the outside world by narrowly over-embedding a network within its social context (Molina-Morales and Martínez-Fernández, 2009). This idea is confirmed by the research on mirror neurons, which appears to indicate that groups with highly hostile interactions with their neighbors tend to have less internal conflict, thus fostering the validation of their own group identity as opposed to that of others (Cohen, Montoya, and Insko, 2006).

Important for peacebuilding work, it seems that the varying power status of groups can affect this dynamic. fMRI studies at MIT have shown that while dialogue between conflicting parties appears to have some positive effects on their capacity for empathy, such effects are highly influenced by the groups' social and political perspectives in relation to each other's perceived status. Both Israeli Jewish and US group members showed positive empathy toward groups of Palestinians and Mexicans during a perspective-taking exercise (i.e., an exercise designed to assist the perception of an alternative point of view, such as that of another individual or group). The empathy of Palestinians and Mexicans did not increase when they were listening to the distress of the Israelis or US groups in relation to bus bombs, lower wages caused by immigrants, etc. Palestinians and Mexicans did however show increased empathy when they perceived that they were attentively listened to by the groups that they perceived to be more powerful (Bruneau and Saxe, 2012). Such findings seem to indicate that the form of dialogue most effective in soliciting empathy differs according to the perceived power asymmetries between the groups and illustrate the need to address, or promise to address, structural societal differences as a complement to, or as part of, effective intergroup dialogue strategies.

Oxytocin—The Bonding Hormone

We are also intrinsically engaged in matters of group bonding through the working of the hormone oxytocin. Oxytocin is a neurohormone whose primary purpose seems to be in stimulating contractions of the uterine wall during childbirth and the milk "let-down" reflex of lactation during nursing (Gordon et al., 2011). However, it also acts on the central nervous system to regulate social behaviors including bonding, trusting, in-group favoritism, empathy, and encouraging generosity (Yang et al., 2013). There are some indicators that the level of oxytocin may be inherited. Kim et al. (2010) observed a genetic variation on the oxytocin receptor gene OXTR at rs53576 between European Americans and Koreans.

The change in oxytocin after a social interaction as measured in a person's blood reflects changes in oxytocin in the brain. Nasally administered oxytocin reduces fear and anxiety (Kirsch et al., 2005) and xenophobic outgroup rejection (Marsh et al., 2017), increases trust (Kosfeld et al., 2005) and empathy (Sheng et al., 2013), and makes you more cooperative, more trustworthy, and more compassionate toward your neighbors (De Dreu et al., 2011). It also reduces the fear of social betrayal in humans and is important for the inhibition of brain regions such as the amygdala as it makes people more likely to cooperate and increases their willingness to accept social risks in interpersonal interactions within their social community.

Unfortunately, this oxycontin-induced cooperation and trust occur intragroup, and not toward groups who are perceived as the out-group. In fact, increased oxytocin, which can help to bond a social group, can lead to more defensive and aggressive behavior toward persons perceived as competing with or being outside of the group (De Dreu et al., 2010, 2011). It can also promote ethnocentric behavior and can increase our suspicion and rejection of those outside our group or the tribe.

The activities of mirror neurons and levels of oxytocin can also increase the level of dehumanization that exists between groups (Haslam, 2006). Historically, dehumanization has always assisted the goals of those who would defeat the other side—its purpose is to enable harm to another group without having to think of them as human. All human societies have prohibitions against harming other humans but not against animals. Somehow the depiction of the other group as akin to animals has historically assisted the colonization of peoples, the persistence of slavery, and acts of genocide. Depicting the others as monkeys, rats, cockroaches, vermin, pigs, etc. has often been essential to furthering a war. In Rwanda Tutsis were referred to as cockroaches, and the Irish were continually depicted by the British media as apes (Wade, 2011). In Israel, the current (2020) deputy defense minister was quoted in an interview as saying, "I don't consider Palestinians as fully human" (Bruneau, 2017).

Such assumptions about our own superiority as a group or nation appear to be universal. A recent study indicated that in every country that was studied (e.g., the United States, England, Denmark, the Netherlands, Spain, Greece, Hungary, Israel, Jordan, and the state of Palestine), people rated at least one group to be at least 15 points lower on the 100-point Ascent dehumanization scale than their own (Kteily et al., 2015). Studies show, for example, that in Europe the degree to which people dehumanize Muslim refugees predicts their support for anti-refugee policies and resistance to refugee settlement, even when accounting for conservatism and prejudice (Bruneau, Kteily, and Laustsen, 2018). A study addressing anti-Muslim rhetoric from the US presidential campaign of 2016 found that the dehumanization of Muslims was strongly associated with the willingness to punish all Muslims for individual acts of terrorism due to the common assumption that out-groups are undifferentiated and therefore collectively responsible for violent actions (Kteily, Hodson, and Bruneau, 2016).

Our almost universal habit of blaming other groups for their actions, but not ourselves, is typical between hostile groups. We usually consider that the violence of our community or nation is excusable and that of the enemies is not. In times of conflict, individuals and groups exhibit a particular tendency to interpret others' behaviors as hostile and their own as more benign (Crick and Dodge, 1996). People are less likely to empathize with the motives of someone outside their group even when both groups are behaving the same way. Hence it is normal to hear groups and nations say that "their" violence is "terrorism" while ours is justified by security needs. This is usually referred to as "attribution bias," and will be dealt with in Chapter 4 of this volume.

Perceptions of Fairness

The discrepancies in feelings of empathy toward groups perceived to be more powerful is also rooted in our bodies' feelings about fairness. Perceived threats in the social environment—when your status, need for certainty, autonomy, relatedness, or sense of fairness is compromised—activate the same neural circuitry in your brain that is activated when you face a physical threat (Rock, 2009). Faced with an apparently unfair deal, the brain's default position is to demand a fair deal.

Even animals appear to have an inherent sense of fairness. In a classic study, two monkeys are placed side by side in separate plexiglass cages, so they can see one another. The first monkey hands the trainer a rock and receives in return a cucumber. Then the second monkey hands the trainer a rock and receives a grape. The first monkey again gives the trainer a rock and receives a cucumber—but after nibbling it, it throws the cucumber back at the trainer and shakes the cage. Every time the scene is repeated, the monkey receiving the cucumber throws it back at the trainer (Dobrin, 2017). The monkey obviously wants the preferable grape for its reward (King, 2014).

Perhaps a sensitivity to fairness in our ancestors was used as a group bonding criterion: fairness meant they were accepted by the tribe and would be protected and given access to resources, whereas unfair treatment put their survival at risk because they could be thrown out or not be fed (Tabibnia and Lieberman, 2007).

The anterior insular cortex of the brain seems to play a central role in such feelings of unfairness, which are experienced as a form of pain (Lack and Bogacz, 2011). In an fMRI experiment, participants were asked to observe fair or unfair players receiving painful electrical shocks. The results of the study showed an interesting difference in terms of the empathy displayed between men and women. The fMRI showed that men's empathy-related neural responses were significantly reduced when they observed unfair players, but this was not the case in women (Kemp and Guastella, 2012).

Such reactions to perceived unfairness also serve group efficacy. The more strongly people identify with a group, the more strongly they will believe that they are the victims of group-based injustice. In addition, they are likely to believe that the group can achieve its goals through collective action (Klavina and Zomeron, 2018). Such discoveries are important to understand when undertaking dialogue or mediation processes—that is, any negotiated agreements need to attend to issues of fairness (even of perceived unfairness) if they are to be sustainable. According to Francis Stewart (2008), horizontal inequalities—those that occur on an identity basis (i.e., people who are excluded/mistreated because of their identity; Stewart, 2008)—are one of the most likely cause of most conflicts today.

Collective Memories

Collective memories play a huge part in the perception of history and of fairness. Collective memory is a "widely shared knowledge of past social events that are collectively constructed through communicative social interactions, which can have a significant impact on our behaviour, feelings, and thoughts" (Garagozov, 2016, p. 28–35).

The purpose of collective memory is to develop and bring meaning to an event and, by extension, to the people it represents. Almost every people, group, or nation has memories of perceived oppressions, which are often passed on to their children in a form of collective identity memory. Such memories are made and maintained through public commemorations and remembrances, through stories, symbols, music, educational curricula, the media, museums, education systems, and political parties, which all continue the collective nature of the group while also often furthering prejudices, conflicts, and persecution (Psaltis, 2016; Volkan, 2009). Volkan (1998) has coined the term "chosen trauma" to refer to such events, which have caused a large group to face drastic losses, feel helpless and victimized by another group, and share a humiliating injury.

Thus there can be a competition for greater victimhood among groups of an ethnic, religious, political, cultural, or language nature can make it more difficult to transform a conflict. Conflicting groups often refer to the nature of their oppression and present their group's history in a positive light and that of other groups in a negative light. Leaders may play a large part in emphasizing such collective memories. Thus a group's history is often viewed as undeserved, unjust, and immoral and one that the group could not prevent (Bar-Tal et al., 2009).

In such a competition for victimhood, it does not seem to matter how long ago such collective memory events took place—for example, biblical events for a Jewish nation according to the Hebrew Bible, the family rifts of 1,400 years ago for Sunni and Shia Muslims, an 850-year occupation by the British in Ireland, the Battle of Kosovo in 1389 for the Serbs, the Armenian "genocide" of 1915, the Nakba of 1948 for Palestinians—such stories, while often dormant in times of relative peace, serve to energize and motivate many current conflicts.

The Threat From Our Own Side

In situations of conflict, the threat of the other side is not always what is most challenging to groups. What is sometimes neglected in peacebuilding work is the fear people feel about their own side and how they are being judged as a loyal or disloyal member of a group. People react more strongly at the neural level to emotional signals from their own in-group members compared to out-group members, and these signals can be validating or threatening (Chiao et al., 2008). Such neural activation has been found in the areas of emotion recognition and inferences of intentions. Neural responses to emotional expressions on Japanese and Caucasian faces, by native Japanese participants in Japan and Caucasian participants in the United States, were examined by Chiao et al. (2008). Obvious neural responses were found by participants in response to in-group members, with participants from both cultures showing greater amygdala activation to faces expressing fear on the part of members of their own cultural groups. Work to address such fears, which can severely limit contact and dialogue, is now happening in some conflicts such as Northern Ireland (Church, Visser, and Johnson, 2002) and Israel (K. Ross, 2017), where it is seen as a useful forerunner to contact and dialogue work between communities.

Given what we know about the importance of bonding and the fear of group betrayal, understanding this fear is critical as it can prevent any collective openness on the part of groups to enter into dialogues with their opponents. If such fear is not addressed, attitudes within group work can be hardened as people consolidate their own group identity and assert their loyalty by displaying views that are nearer to the extreme end of the group's views.

Choosing "Our" Leaders

Leaders are often chosen based on emotional choices, and leaders in search of power rather than peace often use our neural circuitry, as previously noted, and our tendencies to be instinctively fearful of "other" groups to persuade us to vote for them, by priming us to perceive the threat of another group (see Chapter 6 of this volume).

Can Prejudicial Predispositions Change?

Societal environments can moderate attitudes and behavior, and prejudicial tendencies can be mitigated, if not completely erased. One of the most important conclusions from neuroscience research is that the human brain, throughout life, is predisposed to be physically molded, in ongoing ways, by human interactions in contexts that provide for social learning and the rewiring of neural pathways. As we have seen throughout history, our definition of which out-groups are our enemies is socially learned, and throughout most of our group histories such enemies can and do change. This suggests that although our brains are wired for tribalism, they can be (eventually?) rewired to include wider groups through experience and through contexts and institutions that facilitate interaction and tolerance. Some researchers suggest that prejudice toward the other can be decreased because it is due to lack of exposure to other cultures and is not totally hard-wired. People living in more market-integrated societies tend to be more altruistic and tolerant to strangers and more adept at cooperating with them (Buchan et al., 2009). Other evidence for this hypothesis is a decreasing cross-race effect in immigrants that have assimilated to a culture for a few years (Herzmann et al., 2011). Subsequent studies confirmed that assigning people to mixed-race teams can even override racial biases on relatively automatic measures of evaluation (see Van Bavel and Cunningham, 2009) and that the effects of novel group membership can influence perceptual processes within the first few hundred milliseconds of perception (Ratner and Amodio, 2012; Van Bavel et al., 2013).

Another finding in support of this hypothesis is the reversibility of the cross-race effect in adopted ethnic children (Cunningham and Zelazo, 2007). Positive feelings toward people outside of one's group can also result from environmental processes that encourage positive learning about such people (Livingston and Drwecki, 2007). Many studies show that the initial racial bias can be changed through different situational contexts and motivations (Kubota, Banaji, and Phelps, 2012). Familiarity breeds tolerance; for example, differences in amygdala activation have diminished when other-race faces of famous or respected people are viewed, showing that amygdala activation can be controlled through personal beliefs (Marsh, Mendoza-Denton, and Smith, 2010). Also, increasing exposure to other races and cultural ideals helps to suppress the racial bias within the brain circuitry. One study has shown that Asian immigrants who lived in America for an extended period of time did not display a cross-race effect to other American faces, thus implying that exposure to other races decreases such an effect (Herzmann et al., 2011).

Conclusion

Whether we can totally eradicate our tendency to notice and judge others on initial appearance appears doubtful. It is commonplace for peacebuilders to wish for an overarching enemy, perhaps outside of our earthly context, to provide a "safe" target against which humans can unite and forget their differences This hope is a logical one, and based on an accurate perception of human nature. It accords with an understanding of the nature of human groups and the wars between them, and the usefulness of a common enemy around which to rally groups' emotions.

However, we may be reaching a critical point in our world's history. Increasing globalization, boosted by war, environmental threats, and economic and refugee migration, means that we are seeing significant shifts in population diversity in most societies around the world. We are also seeing the internationalization of religious identity wars, which are being played out at a global level. Many threats that the world is facing, such as possible environmental collapse and the operation of worldwide illegal militias, can only be tackled by cooperation between the human population as a whole. Whether we can expand our social circles for such global cooperation is, given our biological history, still in question. Without the development of active social and cultural processes at both local and global levels to encompass such diversification, mass migrations may lead to an increase in the tensions we already see in many parts of the world. Contact with "strangers" against a backdrop of socioeconomic inequalities, which can be exploited by those who wish to breed mistrust and fear for their own personal and group ends, can help create unsettled populations whose hard-wired fears about those who are different to them may result in increasingly violent expression of community tensions.

4

My Truth or Your Truth?

It's not that conservative people are more fearful, it's that fearful people are more conservative.

—Hatemi et al. (2013)

Introduction

In 2015, researchers from the University of York and the University of California, Los Angeles, decided to study how transcranial magnetic stimulation—a noninvasive procedure that uses a metal coil to send pulses to the brain—affected people's approach to social problems (Holbrook et al., 2015). All the participants were politically moderate college undergraduates and were screened to make sure that they held religious convictions before beginning the experiment. As part of the process, participants were asked to rate their belief in the devil, demons, hell, God, angels, and heaven. The participants also read two essays ostensibly written by recent immigrants. One essay was extremely complimentary toward the United States; the other was extremely critical.

The findings revealed that people in whom the targeted brain region was temporarily shut down by transcranial magnetic stimulation reported 32.8 percent less belief in God, angels, or heaven. They were also 28.5 percent more positive in their feelings toward an immigrant who criticized their country. According to the lead author of the report, Dr. Colin Holbrook, "these findings are very striking, and consistent with the idea that brain mechanisms that evolved for relatively basic threat-response functions are repurposed to also produce ideological reactions" ("Belief in God," 2015). Thus, by activating certain regions of the brain, researchers were able to change prejudicial beliefs and even beliefs in God.

In another exercise, ten patients with bilateral damage to the ventromedial prefrontal cortex (vmPFC), ten patients with damage to areas outside the vmPFC, and sixteen medical comparison patients who had experienced

Our Brains at War. Mari Fitzduff, Oxford University Press (2021). © Oxford University Press.
DOI: 10.1093/oso/9780197512654.003.0005

life-threatening (but non-neurological) medical events, completed a series of scales measuring authoritarianism, religious fundamentalism, and specific religious beliefs (Asp et al., 2012). The degree of authoritarianism and religious fundamentalism expressed by those with damage to the vmPFC was significantly higher than the norm for such values. In addition, vmPFC patients reported that their levels of fundamentalism had risen after brain injury.

As I write this book, the social and political institutions of the world seem increasingly fragile and disoriented by the increasing advent of what many see as "false facts" or "fake news," abetted by the use of social media in particular (see Chapter 8 of this volume). Such issues are not new but are now more public and influential because of the apparently infinite communicative power of social media.

However, the juxtaposition of facts to suit our belief systems has always been universal. I have met loyalist paramilitaries in Ireland who believed that the Battle of the Boyne, an icon of Protestant victory that took place in 1690, was enshrined in the Christian Bible. A poll that interviewed 16,063 people from seventeen nations outside the United States to find out who people thought was responsible for the attacks on the World Trade Center in 2001 found that a majority in only nine of the countries believed al-Qaeda carried out the attacks (Allen, 2008). Only 11 percent of Jordanians, 16 percent of Egyptians, 23 percent of Indonesians, and 33 per cent of Mexicans believed it was Al-Qaeda. When asked who they thought was responsible, 43 percent of Egyptians believed it was Israel; 36 percent of Turks believed it was the US government, as did 27 percent the Palestinians. In Britain, 26 percent said they did not know who had carried out the attack, as did 56 percent of the Chinese (Allen, 2008).

Such variance in the beliefs in "facts" is also echoed in countries like the United States, where a survey showed that 55 percent of Americans, and 75 percent of Republicans and evangelicals, believed that Christianity was written into the Constitution and that the founding fathers wanted "One nation under Jesus" (Stone, 2007). A 2015 CNN poll revealed that 20 percent of US citizens still did not believe President Obama was born in the United States: almost 50 percent of Republicans did not believe this. The same poll showed that 29 percent of Americans believed the president was a Muslim, including 43 percent of Republicans (Agiesta, 2015).

How can so many of us be so ignorant—or so blind—to actual facts that seem so important? Generally, it is because it is our emotions that are controlling our beliefs and not our rational intelligence, as many of us would hope or believe. In other words, we often rationalize our beliefs—but usually only after what our guts tell us.

How Do Our Bodies Control Our Beliefs?

Our beliefs in many cases appear to be determined to a large extent not by facts or by the "truth" but by our own bio-tendencies. Many studies have shown that biology and character are inextricably linked. This means that when our physical biology is altered, it can lead to changes in personality, tastes, preferences, perceptions, attention, emotions, attitudes, and behaviors, as well as beliefs.

Twin studies have confirmed the genetic nature of social and political views. In a 2001 study of 195 monozygotic and 141 same-sex dizygotic American twin pairs, researchers observed strong heritability effects for attitudes to capitalism, abortion, education, capital punishment, and organized religion, among other attitude objects (Olson and Jang, 2001).

In 2005, another US twin study examined the attitudes of identical twins regarding twenty-eight social and political issues such as capitalism, trade unions, X-rated movies, abortion, school prayer, divorce, property taxes, and the draft. It compared them to non-identical twins, and it was estimated that genetic factors accounted for 53 percent of the variance (Alford, Funk, and Hibbing, 2005). In a later study using facial electromyography and skin conductance, those who identified as conservatives had larger amygdala structures and those who exhibited a high response to unexpected and unpleasant auditory stimuli were more likely to take conservative positions such as supporting capital punishment, defense spending, the Iraq War, and patriotism (Oxley et al., 2008). Individuals with a lower startle response were more likely to take liberal positions on issues such as supporting foreign aid, gun control, lenient immigration policies, and pacifism.

A larger amygdala volume seems to be positively correlated with dispositional fearfulness as well as with conservatism (Van der Plas et al., 2010). A 2011 study by Kanai et al. found a correlation between differences in political views and differences in brain structures. The researchers performed magnetic resonance imaging (MRI) scans on the brains of ninety volunteer students, who indicated their political orientation ranging from "very liberal" to "very conservative." It was discovered that students who reported more conservative political views tended to have larger amygdalae, while more liberal students tended to have a larger volume of grey matter in the anterior cingulate cortex.

In 2010 a study implicated the gene known as DRD4 in the development of general social/political orientation. Those with a variant of DRD4 called 7R appear to have a predisposition to seeking the new, to listening more closely to the views of friends, and to acquiring a wider circle of friends, thus exposing them to yet more points of view, attitudes, and lifestyles. The research suggests that the development of a liberal disposition requires both a genetic input (the 7R variant) and an environmental one, such as a network of friends, to take effect (Settle et al., 2010). A more recent study by Tusche et al. (2013) confirmed that the ventral striatum was positively correlated with preferential ranking for independent politicians, whereas participants' preferential ranking for the affiliated political parties was reflected in activity in the insula and the cingulate cortex.

Hatemi et al. (2014) have undertaken a study of over 12,000 twin pairs, ascertained from nine different studies conducted in five democracies, sampled over the course of four decades to study the effect of genes on social and political attitudes. They also looked at political attitudes, left–right self-placement, right-wing authoritarianism, life values, economic egalitarianism, individualism versus collectivism, and freedom versus equality. The studies were conducted in Denmark, Australia, Sweden, Hungary, and the United States and were carried out from 1980 to 2011. They found that genetic factors account for a significant amount of the variance in individual differences in ideology across time, location, measures, and populations.

Thus it seems that people who support greater military spending, harsher punishment for criminals, and more restrictive immigration are not doing so not just because they are ignorant or angry about such issues, but because they are more physiologically and psychologically aware of possible negative eventualities. It seems that a more conservative ideology, with its emphasis on tradition, hierarchy, and maintenance of the status quo, provides a better match than liberal or progressive ideology to the feelings of those who feel the prior need to reduce uncertainty and threat (Jost et al., 2017). Thus it make sense that conservatives are more likely to support public policies that would mitigate the dangers they see ahead, in part because their brain patterns lead them to be more cognizant than liberals of such dangers.

Such fears start early in life. Researchers have found that three-year-olds who were rated by teachers as fearful, rigid, indecisive, vulnerable, and inhibited turned out to be more politically conservative as adults. By contrast, three-year-olds who were described as more energetic, resilient, self-reliant, expressive, dominating, and prone to developing close relationships became more liberal in adulthood (Jost and Amodio, 2012).

All of the previous discussion, of course, does not mean that people's specific social or political views are inherited, but it does suggest that a common underlying physical predisposition leads individuals and groups to adopt more conservative bedrock social principles and political ideologies (Ludeke, Johnson, and Bouchard, 2013). Such a predisposition on the part of conservatives to see more dangers ahead, as opposed to liberals who are more likely to see more positive eventualities, may be difficult to change. According to Jonas Kaplan, it can be difficult to change such attitudes as they appear to be intertwined with the natures of our biology (Kaplan, Gimbel, and Harris, 2016).

> Political beliefs are like religious beliefs in the respect that both are part of who you are and important for the social circle to which you belong. To consider an alternative view, you would have to consider an alternative version of yourself. (Jonas Kaplan, quoted in "Hard-Wired," 2016)

Group Belief Binding/Blinding?

What is the evolutionary purpose of varying beliefs such as those previously noted? As we have seen in Chapter 3 of this volume, our views as part of a group are usually a groupthink (i.e., based on group traditions rather than on fact-checking). They are what Haidt calls "groupish" which means that we usually approve of what we think, or what are told is good for our group (Runciman, 2012). We inherit most of our beliefs, perhaps as a legacy of what helped our ancestors survive. Our attachment to group belonging, and its attendant beliefs, may have helped groups in the past to win the societal competition for group-level survival and to gain from what has been described as "parochial altruism" (Yamagishi and Mifune, 2016).

It appears that almost any ideological framework, whether religious, cultural, or social, can be used to strengthen group bonds and serve as a binding factor. Religious beliefs are a clear example of such a binding process, given that they remain the most dominant group belief system: 84 percent of the world's population belongs to some form of organized religion (Pew

Research Center, 2012). Our beliefs can be very powerful motivators for individual and collective action, including violent action. Almost all forms of religion—Christianity, Buddhism, Islam, Hinduism, Judaism—have served throughout history, and many still do today, to provide not only meaning and comfort to many but also frameworks of belief that justify exclusion and violence (see Chapter 5 of this volume).

Most people are biased toward beliefs that fit well with, or reinforce, their existing beliefs or values, or their particular individual or group context. Once adopted, the beliefs often continue to be held regardless of their coherence with reality. Groups will often hold on to such beliefs regardless of rational challenges to them. Thus the "truths" felt at, for example, Trump rallies will matter far more to many Trump supporters than those expounded in newspapers, by other politicians, or by academics.

It is important to note that functions served by group beliefs, such as a sense of solidarity and collectiveness and a meaning to one's existence, often matter more than the substance of such beliefs. Those of us who have tried to have theological, moral, or social discussions with religious or social fundamentalists have usually found how unsuccessful such a rational exchange process can be. It seems that the reality is that many of our reactions to information are not rational but rather automatic and emotional, and in fact are actually set in motion before any conscious thought. (Mooney, 2012b).

We All Think We Have the Truth

The neural infrastructure built up around maintaining our "truths"—our ideological righteousness—is enormous. It appears that such a predisposition, as well as confirmation bias—that is, the adjustment of our thinking to fit what we want to believe—is an essential part of an evolutionary adaptation as a built-in feature to our survival. Since these processes occur automatically, in regions of our brain that are generally inaccessible to consciousness, we are often subject to their effects whether we like it or not. Most of us, as psychologists Lee Ross and Andrew Ward (1996) said, are "naïve realists" who believe that we alone see the world objectively, whereas those who disagree with us are often seen as inherently irrational. These "bias blind spots" appear to be part of a consequence of having a human brain that is designed to operate efficiently (Bruneau, 2016).

Once we are part of a group, a process called *deindividuation* can take place. This means that people often give up their personal identity and beliefs to belong to a group and to gain from such membership. Usually, on joining a group, an individual's attitude changes in the direction of the group norm. Previous beliefs may be discarded or changed to fit with new ones. Once group beliefs become sacrosanct, members often lose their ability (and their freedom) to think rationally about them. This is helped by the fact that, once our views have been formed, we have a tendency to see and find evidence in support of them and ignore evidence that challenges them. Scientifically fact-based arguments often do not work to change people's beliefs. When asked to choose between accepting the views of an expert (such as on global warming) and being a good member of a tribe, relying on anecdotes they have heard from someone they trust, or relying on personal experiences, the latter is more important to many people (Achenbach, 2015; Kysar and Salzman, 2005).

In a functional MRI (fMRI) study, Westen et al. (2006) showed that when faced with logical contradictions to deeply held beliefs, people may feel negative emotions, but there is no actual increase in their reasoning cortex. Another fMRI study, by Harris, Sheth, and Cohen (2008), showed that when faced with statements that contradicted their deeply held beliefs, participants showed a negative emotional response akin to "disgust," while statements that confirmed beliefs were greeted with positive responses. Most of us do all that we can to protect our group beliefs by watching media sources such as Fox News or MSNBC or by reading the *New York Times* or the *Washington Times*, the *Daily Telegraph* or *Guardian*, *Haaretz* or *Jerusalem Post*, etc., often to solidify what we believe. Even when watching the same media coverage of their conflicts, conflicting groups think it is biased against them (Perloff, 2015).

Motivated Reasoning

Motivated reasoning is sometimes termed *rational irrationality* (Huemer, n.d.). This does not mean that an individual deliberately chooses to believe something they knows to be false, but rather that people allow themselves to be more easily influenced by emotional appeals and their own cognitive biases when making decisions. For rational irrationality to exist, certain beliefs must be appealing to people for reasons other than their truth value. Huemer (n.d.) identifies some possible sources of bias, for example *self-interested bias,* in which people hold beliefs that, if accepted, would benefit themselves or the group with whom they identify; *self-image constructors,* which means that people prefer to hold beliefs that best fit with the images of themselves that they want to adopt and to project; beliefs that are *tools of social bonding*—that is, people prefer to hold the beliefs of the people with whom they want to associate; and *coherence bias* beliefs that fit well with or reinforce their existing beliefs. So important is it to believe what we want to believe that we even have the capacity to deceive ourselves—to come to believe what we say. Thus we can say with conviction, for example, that there has always been global warming but it is not caused by humans or smoking is not bad for you—"My grandfather smoked all his life and he lived till ninety" (Livingstone Smith, 2007)—not even knowing that such reasoning is likely to be motivated reasoning.

Given the extent of motivated reasoning, it has been suggested that we have been reasoning about reasoning incorrectly, because we have misunderstood what its original purpose was. Mercier and Sperber (2012) have suggested that human reason did not evolve as a device for getting at an objective truth. Rather, its purpose is to facilitate selective arguing within groups to get at the "wisdom of the crowd." Mooney (2012a) agrees with this, noting that there would have been a survival value to a process that would have helped people to benefit from an airing of different views, so that their strengths and weaknesses could be debated. Thus the process of arguing was of survival value, rather than the truth itself.

While this may have been a valuable approach in hunter-gatherer times, in these days, when it is becoming possible for almost seven billion of us to state our own truth, the skill of community discussion on where to track animals and find food and safety is likely to be a mismatch in terms of today's need for large-group consensus.

Attribution errors are an extension of motivated reasoning. One of the established findings of the social psychological field has been that people tend to explain others' behavior as arising from their personality, while neglecting situational causality (L. Ross, 1977). In other words, we tend to try to find justifications for our own beliefs and actions when something bad happens or is done by us, but not for the same actions by other people or groups. We often feel and say that such actions are their fault, not ours: for example, their violence is terrorism; ours is justified by security needs. In Ireland this was often called the "whataboutery" argument, as in "So we may have done wrong in killing ten people who were peacefully watching a game of football in a pub, or butchering an innocent bystander, but look what they did to us yesterday, last month, 100 years ago, etc."

Uncertainty Avoidance

As we have seen, people genetically differ in their dislike of ambiguity and their need for certainty. At one end of the spectrum, some people appear to have genetically greater sensitivity and dislike of uncertainty and a greater need for order, structure, and clear beliefs in their lives—differences that can be observed from birth. At the other end are people who are genetically more open to new things and to new experiences that require cognitive complexity. They can better tolerate nuances of belief and certainty. One of the measurements for this is called *integrative complexity*. This reflects the capacity of a person or society to tolerate uncertainty and ambiguity within a society, as well as their capacity for accepting new information or ideas. It also reflects a people or group's ability to be flexible in considering change, as well as their capacity for cognitive nuances (Suedfeld, Leighton, and Conway, 2006). A lack of such integrative complexity can be a problem in trying to achieve peace agreements. Research shows that low integrative complexity is often associated with reduced effectiveness in resolving conflicts and also with increased other-directed attributions of blame (Sillars and Parry, 1982). In addition, people with lower levels of integrative complexity are more likely to resort to competitive actions like war, and more likely to use violence when frustrated, whereas individuals with higher integrative complexity may have enhanced chances for successful negotiation and nonviolent conflict resolution (Conway, Suedfeld, and Tetlock, 2001).

One of the key differences between contexts with weak and strong societal uncertainty avoidance is in their establishment of law and rules. Cultures with low uncertainty avoidance have fewer and often somewhat more general laws and rules, whereas countries with high uncertainty avoidance establish many and precise laws and rules (Hofstede, 1997). Thus, a country with a high uncertainty avoidance score is usually a very rule-oriented society and follows well-defined and established laws, regulations, and controls. A low uncertainty-avoidance score points to a society that is less concerned about ambiguity and uncertainty and has more tolerance for variety, experimentation, and risk-taking.

Another factor related to uncertainty avoidance is a person or group's level of *need for closure* (Kruglanski and Webster, 1996). Such a need describes an individual's desire for a firm answer to a question and an aversion to ambiguity. A person with a high need for closure tends to use a piece of information that suits them and then freeze, refusing to consider new information. Studies show that conservatives tend to have a greater need for closure than do liberals, which is to be expected in light of the strong relationship between liberalism and openness. Panno et al. (2018) investigated the need for cognitive closure as a predictor of political orientation and found a strong connection between them.

This desire for certainty also informs our perspectives on leaders. We prefer our leaders to speak with certainty about issues we are concerned about—often irrespective of the substance of their arguments. Leaders who express hesitation, or even endorse the value of consultation, can be anathema to us. Our need is for them to be clear and strong, particularly if we are afraid. For many conservatives, uncertainty or indecisiveness can be seen as a weakness (see Chapter 6 of this volume).

Right versus Wrong?

Mutually agreed value systems also assist shared values and cooperation. It seems that morality is nature's assistance to the problem of cooperation within groups, enabling individuals with competing interests to coordinate their social interactions as well as suppressing selfish or aggressive behavior (de Waal, 2006). Moral beliefs, in tandem with other beliefs, are mostly intuitive rather than rational in everyday use. Haidt (2012, p. 47) has developed a social intuitionist model of moral judgment, which suggests that moral judgment is mostly based on automatic processes—moral intuitions—rather than on conscious reasoning. He suggests that people engage in reasoning largely to find evidence to support what they instinctively feel and that they then make a rational-sounding justification for that feeling Critcher, Inbar, and Pizarro (2013).

For most people, moral reasoning is usually generated only after a belief has been assumed instinctively. This is why people are often inconsistent in the way they apply their values to their political beliefs (e.g., citing the value of life, denying abortion rights while at the same time supporting capital punishment; Critcher et al., 2009). They argue that this difference is rooted in the distinct ways that liberals and conservatives represent political issues. They suggest that conservatives' higher need for closure leads them to represent issues in terms of salient, accessible values. "Although this may lead conservatives" attitudes to be more situationally malleable under some circumstances, such shifts do serve to protect an absolutist approach to one's moral values and help conservatives to deny the comparability of potentially inconsistent positions' (Critcher et al., 2009, p. 181). Their studies suggest that while liberals and conservatives respond similarly to considerations of harm/care and fairness, conservatives respond more strongly to considerations of in-group, authority, and purity (Cole Wright and Baril, 2011).

Such differences in value prioritizations present significant challenges for the peacebuilding field. As shown in Haidt and Joseph's (2004) moral foundation theory, for some people, such as those on the more "liberal" side, care for others and fairness to others—including those beyond our own loyalty groups, such as immigrants—are priority values, and they often see the need to have such values incorporated into a government's social structures. For other groups, sanctity, authority, liberty, and order are values that matter more than the "fairness" and "caring" exemplified by "big government." Such value differences affect ideas about peacebuilding, the role of governments, wealth distribution, and the role of leaders and are the source of political and social differences in many parts of the world today (Zambakari, 2017).

Differences in such values can affect the making of peace agreements, post-conflict institution building, and agreed processes of democracy and good governance, all of which need to be balanced in relation to differing value systems on the part of participants and constituencies. Groups sometimes have distinctive moral or value commitments, such as religious ones, that other groups don't recognize as authoritative. An understanding of the basic differences among groups involved in peace processes is therefore critical in helping to understand and appreciate what underlies many international and societal conflicts and what is essential to fostering sustainable agreements between groups.

System Justification

System justification is the idea that many people are motivated to defend and bolster existing social, economic, and political arrangements, not necessarily because they are right, but because doing so addresses their basic psychological needs, including their need to attain and retain certainty and order (Jost, Gaucher, and Stern, 2015). Many researchers have observed that system-justification scores were associated with greater bilateral amygdala volume (Nam et al., 2018). It is an important aspect of conservatism insofar as it involves a resistance to change, a maintenance of the status quo, and a justification of inequality (Jost, Nosek, and Gosling, 2008). Researchers have found that system justification is a potentially strong motivator of human behavior, because it addresses fundamental human needs to reduce uncertainty, threat, and social discord (Jost, Ledgerwood, and Hardin, 2008a). Rationalization of the status quo is often associated with short-term feelings of comfort. On an emotional level, system justification makes conservative people feel better, happier and more satisfied than liberals with the status quo through, for example, an acceptance of inequality (Butz, Kieslich, and Bless, 2017). The problem for peacebuilders is that such acceptance can mitigate proactivity toward remedies addressing inequality and thereby affect the development of institutions that can address such inequalities and potentially end a war and begin to sustain peace.

Such ideas suggest that countries that are home to diverse ethnic or religious groups, whose outlooks are characterized by strong uncertainty avoidance, tend to be more prone to intergroup tensions, given their decreased potential for social change and their reluctance to address issues of inequality. Given such defensiveness, Jost (2017) has noted that "system justification can lead us to deny and excuse aspects of our society—such as the ever-widening gap between rich and poor and the damage we are doing to the natural environment, to take just two very salient and worrisome examples—that we ought to confront sooner rather than later" (see also Bridge and Voss, 2014).

Memories and Beliefs

All wars are fought twice, the first time on the battlefield, the second time in memory.

—Viet Thanh Nguyen

Our memories are notoriously faulty—they often reframe and edit events to fit our current situation, conflating the past and present to suggest a story that suits what we need to believe today. Our memories are like a network that can retrieve ideas according to our purposes and our emotions and thus determine what the conscious mind has available to work with—and to argue with.

> Your memory reframes and edits events to create a story to fit your current world. It's built to be current. . . . It is like a wily time traveler, plucking fragments of the present and inserting them into the past. In terms of accuracy, it is no video camera. Rather, the memory rewrites the past with current information, updating your recollections with new experiences to aid survival. (Bridge and Voss, 2014, https://www.sciencedaily.com/releases/2014/02/140204185651.htm)
>
> Thus, memory tends to be adaptive in nature and so can be reconstructed each time we revisit an event. It appears that in our everyday lives we construct stories about our lives and endow meaning and causality between different events that happen to us. Thus we understand ourselves by creating our autobiographies from memories that are frequently the products of distortion. (Schacter, Guerin, and St Jacques, 2011; also see McAdams, 2013)

In other words, as Hibbing, Smith, and Alford (2014, p. 241) have said, "if the facts get in the way of your preferred worldview, just unwittingly 'misremember' the facts."

Collective memories are the set of memories that are shared among a group (Brown, Kouri, and Hirst, 2012). They constitute "a shared set of representations of the past based on a common identity to a group" (Licata and Klein, 2005, p. 243). Collective memories, particularly in situations of conflict, are almost always biased and politicized. Their purpose is to bind groups together and help create and sustain group identities through collective memory distortion that ranges from "active forms of forgetting" (Ricoeur, 2006) through the careful erasure of archival sources and "pacts of silence" (Ben-Ze'Evev, Ginio, and Winter, 2010), all of which can help create "collective amnesia" (K. Walsh, 2001).

Societies in conflict all over the world engage in collective memory distortion when tensions arise. They can newly revile an old enemy and reinvent memories of events in a way that puts their case and their side in a positive light, often denying or dismissing atrocities they may have themselves committed. Depending on their specific aims, people will choose particular historical events, moments, or figures to strengthen their arguments or champion their goals. This means that whenever a specific social identity is salient, individuals may remember some historical events or periods in a specific way and attach to them evaluations and emotions that are shared at least to some extent by other in-group members but may or may not be shared by out-group members (Figueiredo et al., 2017). Interestingly, the very same past may be used by different political actors to achieve quite different aims. Such redesigned history is regularly mobilized by politicians, activists, or the media to justify, contextualize, or legitimize ideological claims or political and societal standpoints.

Beliefs and Party Politics

In 2006, a study by Drew Westen and his colleagues suggested that there were differences between US Republicans and Democrats in how they think about political questions (Westen, Blagov, Harenski, Kilts, and Hamann, 2006). In a subsequent article, Hatemi et al. (2008) found that genetics plays a significant role in shaping the strength of a person's party identification. Neither study was about definitive party affiliation. It appears that there are no genes that make people be, for example, US Democrats or Republicans or members of British Labour or Conservative political parties, any more than there are genes that make people believe in Christianity or Islam or Hinduism. However, there are differences in their emotional and cognitive scaffolding from which they approach political challenges. This means that social or political prejudices can be sustained by basic-level neurocognitive structures whose expression is guided by people's personal goals and existing social expectations of particular intergroup settings (Amodio, 2014). Most recently, other researchers have concluded that the heritability of party identification depends on the context, in particular in situations of increasing partisan polarization (Fazekas and Littvay, 2015).

As we have noted, personal needs for order, structure, and cognitive closure are positively associated with resistance to change, acceptance of inequality, system justification, political conservatism, and right-wing orientation (Federico et al., 2013). These tendencies will play out in terms of people's party politics. Thus studies have found that Republicans used their right amygdala, the part of the brain associated with the body's fight-or-flight system, when making risk-taking decisions, while Democrats tended to show greater activity in their left insula, an area that is associated with self-awareness and social awareness (Schreiber et al., 2013). Schreiber et al.

claim that their study suggested an 82.9 percent accuracy rate in predicting whether a person is a Democrat or Republican through the study of amygdala reactions. It also suggests that such reaction positively predicts a participant's snap decision to vote for someone based solely on appearance, a phenomenon that was observed across cultures.

Not Just Genes and Brains

A meta-study (Hatemi et al., 2014) summarized all reported twin and kinship studies that provided estimates of genetic and environmental influences on political traits from 1974 to 2012. The study looked at the aggregate effect of all genetic influences, shared or common environmental influences, and unique environmental influences, which included idiosyncratic experiences. The findings suggested that while genes undoubtedly matter for the development of political attitudes, individual common variants will have small effects on ideology. It is not therefore that

> an individual is born with a fixed attitudinal disposition, but rather all those elements of the individual's psychological architecture, including perception, emotion, cognition, reasoning, affect, affiliation, and countless other attentional categories, are to varying degrees a function of inherited and developed biological mechanisms. These mechanisms play an important role in the probabilities of selecting into, experiencing, interpreting, and responding to social experiences. (Hatemi and McDermott, 2016, p. 333)

For instance, it appears that education has a large influence on out-group attitudes, with more highly educated people displaying more supportive attitudes toward out-groups (Hatemi et al., 2013). Exactly how much our personal genetics influences our attitudes and behavior is still a major research question.

Fundamentalist Beliefs

The term "fundamentalist" was originally used within the United States to designate a particular strand of American Protestantism that believed absolutely in the eternal "truths" of the Christian Bible, as opposed to more flexible Protestants who believed that their understanding of the Bible could be adjusted in light of new information offered by science. There is a continuum with absolute dependency on a set of clear beliefs at one end and flexibility in terms of beliefs at the other. While there are fundamentalists within all the major faith systems (e.g., Christianity, Buddhism, Islam, and Hinduism), they are usually a minor section of such adherents. Also, many common fundamentalist beliefs relate to socialist or market-based principles.

Fundamentalist beliefs can be harmless to both individuals and society unless they infringe others' rights, and/or motivate people to violence (see Chapter 5 of this volume). They are a version of believing that is positioned far to the non-negotiable side. Fundamentalists like clear and agreed "truths," which are (they hope) unchangeable and nonnegotiable irrespective of the contexts in which they live. They want and need a simple and clear framework of meaning and ownership of the truth. They have little or no tolerance for complexity or nuances of belief, and they allow little room for nuanced or favorable interpretations of the out-group. They will use many of the previously noted processes such as motivated reasoning, system justification, uncertainty avoidance, moral certainty, proclaimed ownership of the truth, and fear of out-groups. According to Kruglanski (2014), they paint

> a Manichean worldview characterized by sharp dichotomies and clear choices; a world of good versus evil, saints versus sinners, order versus chaos; a pure universe in black and white admitting no shades of gray. A fundamentalist ideology establishes clear contingencies between actions and consequences; it offers a future that is predictable and controllable.

Such groups often go to extraordinary lengths to avoid exposure to differing beliefs. Other groups than their own are often designated as less than human, and their sense of their own specialness is often validated. There are also extreme versions of in-group control and an exaggerated intolerance of norm violations (Kossowska et al., 2016, pp. 390–391).

Cynics?

Some researchers assert that determining social/political tendencies from fMRI data is overreaching that technology's capacity. They express concerns about the ability of researchers to distinguish genetic from environmental effects, given that these are interactive in nature (Charney and English, 2012). And, as we have seen, contexts also matter a lot. Thus, a study of survivors who were highly impacted by the 9/11 attack on the New York World Trade Center found that three times as many survivors reported becoming more politically conservative in the eighteen months following the attack, regardless of partisan identification (Bonanno and Jost, 2006).

For some researchers, this division of differences into traditionalist/liberal dimensions in not multidimensional enough, and in their fMRI studies they have identified three different patterns of brain activation that they believe correlate with individualism, conservatism, and radicalism (Zamboni et al., 2019). They believe that these three independent dimensions explain the variability of a set of statements expressing political/social beliefs. Each dimension was reflected in a distinctive pattern of neural activation: individualism in the medial prefrontal cortex and in the temporoparietal junction of the brain, conservatism in the dorsolateral prefrontal, and radicalism in the ventral striatum and posterior cingulate areas.

Conclusion

No doubt the arguments about how much our belief systems are determined by our bio-predispositions will continue. However, it is useful to note that the research is conclusive about there being such an effect. It is therefore useful for the peacebuilder to note that innate predispositions and their group effects can make it harder, or sometimes easier, to conduct the peacebuilding work that is necessary to achieve an agreement that can help a society—or the globe—better function without violence. Such work will not be easy or quick. As Hibbing et al. (2014, p. 23) have noted, "altering a [genetic] predisposition is like turning a supertanker; it usually takes concerted force for an extended period of time, but it can be done."

5

The Lure of Extremism

What inspires the most uncompromisingly lethal actors in the world
today is not so much the Qur'an or religious teachings. It's a thrilling
cause that promises glory and esteem. Jihad is an egalitarian, equal-
opportunity employer: fraternal, fast-breaking, glorious, cool—and
persuasive.

—Atran (2015)

Introduction

They went to school together, studied martial arts together and,
on occasion, chatted over cups of coffee. Yet when civil war swept
the former Yugoslavia, enveloping the Bosnian town of Kozarac in
the spring of 1992, Dusko Tadic, an ethnic Serb, turned on Emir
Karabasic, a Bosnian Muslim. According to the testimony of 50
witnesses the former bar owner raped, tortured and murdered
Muslim and Croat civilians. No single offense though, approached
the savagery of what he did to Karabasic: In the garage of an "ethnic
cleansing" concentration camp near Kozarac, Tadic allegedly forced
a prisoner to bite off Karabasic's testicles, then allowed his former
neighbor to bleed to death. (Rogers, 1995)

Unfortunately, extreme violence to perpetrate wars and to pursue resource
and political divisions is ubiquitous and has been used since time immemo-
rial by most parties to a conflict. It has been estimated that over 160 million
people have died in wars during the twentieth and twenty-first centuries
(Scaruffi, 2009). The vast majority of these were killed by states, and not
by illegal militias (i.e., those that are not sanctioned by a state). Such illegal
militias are variously called "terrorists," "combatants," "freedom fighters,"
etc., depending on the context and the speaker. The term "violent extremism"
is now used by many agencies to enhance the contextual nature of the term

Our Brains at War. Mari Fitzduff, Oxford University Press (2021). © Oxford University Press.
DOI: 10.1093/oso/9780197512654.003.0006

(Futures without Violence, 2017). The Global Terrorism Index noted 163 such groups in 2019 (Institute for Economics and Peace, 2019).

According to the Global Terrorism Index, the total number of deaths from terrorism is minuscule compared to those of "normal" wars. Terrorism deaths declined for the fourth consecutive year in 2020, falling by 15.2 percent to **13,826**, with most of these deaths occurring in Afghanistan, Iraq, and Syria. Accirding to the New America Foundation, jihadists killed 94 people inside the United States between 2005 and 2015; 301,797 people in the United States were shot dead during the same period (Anderson, 2017). However, although terrorism poses only a tiny risk to people, it tends to be a major fear factor for many in the United States. At least part of this bias is probably due to the uncertainty factor of terrorism: the unpredictability of such attacks, and the emotions around them, tend to result in the risk being seen as much greater than the risk of a car death. In addition, tactics used by terror groups, such as beheading, torture, and mass civilian bombings, have rightly horrified many. In fact, no strategies or tactics used by those who are usually termed "terrorists" have not at some stage been used by legal entities. The difference is that illegal militias often take great care to ensure that their horrific acts can be seen by the world through both regular and social media. Evidence seems to suggest that increasing the visibility of acts of terror can diffuse such fear widely and make it disproportionate to the reality (Holman, Garfin, and Cohen Silver, 2019).

The Normality of Violent Extremists

Contrary to what many leaders say, people who use illegal violence to further their political or religious ends are not generally psychopaths or even mentally ill. Crenshaw's comprehensive 1981 work on the causes of terrorism, which was based on decades of observations with a variety of groups ranging from nineteenth-century Russian anarchists to Irish, Israeli, Basque, and Algerian nationalists, found nothing to suggest that such people were any different to the psychological norm. In fact, the outstanding common characteristic of individual terrorists, Crenshaw concluded, is their normality. In 2004, Sageman examined the motivations of 172 jihadist terrorists as revealed primarily in court documents. His conclusions, drawn from decades of jail interviews and psychological studies, showed that terrorism is not reducible to either ideological or religious motivations, nor to personality disorders.

More recent studies on militant members of groups such as the Fuerzas Armadas Revolucionarias de Colombia (FARC) in Colombia, Islamic State of Iraq and Syria (ISIS) in the Middle East, or the Irish Republican Army (IRA) in Ireland note that most members show no signs of psychopathology (Decety, Pape, and Workman, 2018).

Disturbing as it may be, individuals who become radicalized and involve themselves with terrorist organizations are, on the whole, ordinary people with typically functioning brains. Most are not psychopaths, and with perhaps the exception of "lone wolf" terrorists, they are not especially likely to have psychiatric diagnoses (Horgan, 2014). Although researchers have found two genes—monoamine oxidase and cadherin 13—that, when mutated, appeared to correlate with violent, even homicidal behavior, no connection between these naturally occurring regulators and the behavior of violent extremists has been made (Tiihonen et al., 2015).

Why Do People Join Violent Extremist Movements?

Many studies across ideologies and time describe the multifaceted nature of radicalization, and its relationship to its environmental context. The Tamil Tigers/Sri Lanka, IRA/Ireland, ETA/Basque Country, Naxalites/India, Maoists/Nepal, and the many past and present Middle Eastern and African jihadist groups offer varying motives to explain their membership of their groups. Even within apparently simple identity groups, motivations will vary widely; for example, jihadist group members have differing stated motivations depending on whether they are from the Western world, Asia, Africa, or the Middle East.

Rarely about Beliefs

It is sometimes contended that people convert or deepen their particular social, cultural, or religious beliefs, which leads them to use violence to implement such beliefs in policy and practice. However, many researchers assert that ideology is usually not the primary motivating factor (Sageman, 2004). As Chapter 4 of this volume has shown, beliefs are more like the clothes that people put on to belong to a particular group and to carry out particular actions: their beliefs can and often do provide justifications for their membership of such groups. Testosterone-driven young men looking to be heroic are not, by and large, often involved in political or theological discussions or always poring over sacred texts of the Koran, the Bible, or Marx and Engels before they decide to join a militia group. Rather such texts will help to provide a rationalization for the radicals' violence but are often a quite minor part of their stories (Roy, 2017). According to leaked Islamic State of Iraq and the Levant (ISIL) records containing details of more than 4,000 foreign recruits, while most of the fighters were well educated, 70 percent stated that they had only basic knowledge of Islam (Roy, 2017).

Many locals in the Middle East join militia groups for economic benefits. Research conducted in Somalia showed that 27 percent of respondents joined al-Shabaab for economic reasons; 15 percent mentioned religious reasons, and 13 percent were forced to join (Botha and Abdile, 2014). My own research in Northern Ireland showed mixed motives for joining the IRA, which was the nationalist militia, and loyalist militias such as the Ulster Defence Association and the Ulster Volunteer Force. The first motivation was a long-standing family heritage of opposition to the occupation of Ireland by the British. The second was a response to an incident in which family or friends had been injured or killed. The third—mostly among Loyalist groups—was a desire to have a respected role as a man in their community, which was particularly important for those who were unemployed (Fitzduff, 1989).

Such motivations on the part of extremists can change. For example, due to the current profit- and greed-based possibilities of being part of the Naxalite Maoist insurgency, the movement has moved far from ideology and its principles of armed revolution (Prasad, 2015). While the FARC movement claimed to be fighting for the rights of the poor in Colombia and to provide social justice through communism, it eventually turned to funding its operations through kidnapping and ransom, illegal mining, extortion, and the production and distribution of illegal drugs (McDermott, 2012).

In 2008, a classified briefing note on radicalization, prepared by MI5's behavioral science unit, suggested that, far from being religious zealots, a large number of those involved in terrorism do not practice their faith regularly (Travis, 2008). According to criminologist Andrew Silke (quoted in Byrne, 2017), who conducted many interviews with imprisoned jihadists, motives on the part of Western recruits are also often confused:

> When I ask them why they got involved, the initial answer is ideology. But if I talk to them about how they got involved, I find out about family fractures, what was happening at school and in their personal lives, employment discrimination, yearnings for revenge for the death toll of Muslims.

For many recruits from the West, religious fervor often arises outside of the usual faith structures and is adopted either not long before terrorists move into action or soon after an individual has joined an organization (Roy, 2017). Would-be jihadist recruits Yusuf Sarwar and Mohammed Ahmed ordered *Islam for Dummies* and *The Koran for Dummies* on Amazon just before they set out from Birmingham to join ISIL in Syria (Hasan, 2014). According to Roy (2017), it appears that the fascination that the Islamic State holds for thousands of French youths "is not about the radicalisation of Islam, but the Islamisation of radicality."

Local Middle Eastern recruits, on the other hand, are often driven by factors such as a sense of injustice, the constant need for security in conflict situations, and the need to survive, often by belonging tightly to a particular militia group. Many recruits within such groups change allegiances as more successful or better-paying groups emerge. Within Syria, many of the recruits are purely economic actors, who are recruited with offers of good salaries, health insurance, and benefits paid to their families if they are killed in battle (Byrne, 2017). Particulars of belief are often secondary to shifting group allegiances. Byrne notes that "the local ISIS rank and file is often down-to-earth: disenfranchised people struggling to eke out a living for their families in war zones . . . women . . . had encouraged their husbands and sons to join ISIS in order to get better family living quarters."

Of course, many people do not get the chance to volunteer themselves for conflicts—they are forced into joining. A 2004 Human Rights Watch report noted that UNICEF had documented 3,516 cases of underage recruitment since the signing of the ceasefire agreement in Sri Lanka in 2002 and estimated that the Tamil Tigers had more than 5,000 child soldiers in its ranks, some as young as ten.

Not the Poorest

While poverty and economic exclusion has often been cited as a cause for recruits to join militias, they are often not the poorest, the most humiliated, or the least integrated (Roy, 2017). Many of those who are attracted to violent extremism are relatively well-educated, come from affluent backgrounds, but are "frustrated achievers" in that their talents are not sufficiently utilized within their societal context. A study of the biographies of 335 deceased Palestinian suicide bombers discovered that only 16 percent of the sample had an income rated below the poverty line, while 31 percent of Palestinians as a whole are classified as impoverished. No fewer than 96 percent had achieved a high school diploma, while 65 percent had benefited from at least some form of higher education. In contrast, only 51 percent of the Palestinian population at large have a high school education and only 15 percent have some higher education. Of the studied terrorists, 94 percent had employment, as opposed to only 69 percent of the broader Palestinian population. Thus the evidence suggests that Palestinian suicide bombers tend to be actually less deprived than the average Palestinian (Benmelech and Berrebi, 2007).

Justice Motivation

The greater the political inequality of minority groups within a state, the more terrorism a state is likely to face. "Justice motivation"—the capacity for perceiving injustice toward oneself and one's group—often plays a central role in the narratives of violent terrorists. As we have seen in Chapter 4 of this volume, the perception that one's group has been treated unfairly and is a victim of injustices, whether political, economic, or religious, is believed to play a critical role in motivating anger and acts of terrorism (Decety and Yoder, 2017). Such perceptions of victimization can be an important turning point in recruitment to violence (Pemberton and Aarten, 2018). For instance, Palestinian youths who felt as though their group had received unjust treatment reported greater support for religiopolitical aggression (Victoroff et al., 2011). Perceived injustice was also a determinant of turning toward a radical belief system in young Dutch Muslim youths (Doosje, Loseman, and van den Bos, 2013; Victoroff et al., 2011). It is thus not a surprise that such victimization narratives are heavily used in the propaganda materials produced and distributed by violent extremist organizations in an effort to garner recruits.

While concern for justice is a part of human nature and emerges early in childhood, it seems that some individuals are more highly sensitive to injustice than others (Decety and Yoder, 2016). Interestingly, such justice sensitivity has been associated with brain activation in regions thought to relate to neural responses in the cortex—that is, the part of the brain involved in executive functioning, working memory, and response selection—on the part of participants who were asked to rate scenarios that depicted interpersonal assistance or harm as either morally good or bad (Decety et al., 2018). "Sacred values differ from material or instrumental ones by incorporating moral beliefs that drive action in ways dissociated from prospects for success. Across the world, people believe that devotion to core values (such as the welfare of their family and country or their commitment to religion, honor, and justice) is, or ought to be, absolute and inviolable. Such values outweigh other values, particularly economic ones" (Atran, Axelrod, and Davis, 2007, p. 1039). Such values are present in most conflicts that are about identity issues. In Morocco, people's willingness to engage in militant jihad, and its associated sacrifices, was especially pronounced in individuals who considered Sharia a sacred value (Atran, Sheikh, and Gomez, 2014). Similarly, Israelis and Palestinians who were presented with hypothetical Israeli–Palestinian peace deals were strongly opposed to deals that just included material incentives, but their opposition decreased when their opponents were willing to make symbolic concessions relating to their sacred values (Ginges et al., 2007). A neuroimaging study has confirmed this: the sacred values that participants were unwilling to sacrifice in exchange for material gain were associated with activation in the ventrolateral prefrontal cortex and left temporoparietal junction (Berns et al., 2012).

Such felt injustices need not be about one's own life; they can concern the sufferings of others. The fact that illegal militia members say that they are motivated by the "suffering" experienced by others who were formerly colonized or victims of racism or US aggression suggests that it is not a sense of impoverishment that drives extreme violence, but often a cognitive and empathetic attachment with the dispossessed (McAllister and Schmid, 2011, p. 250). Such an attachment can explain not only the attraction of jihadism among the middle and professional classes in their respective countries but also the prominence of the sons and daughters of middle- and upper-class parents among Western fighters (Decety et al., 2018).

Given that justice motivations are part of the stories of many recruits to violent extremism, it is important to address such structural causes in the lives of those who are socially excluded, or perceive themselves to be so, to diminish the power of such exclusion as a motivating factor. Atran et al. (2014) found that the profiles of jihadists who seek justice for their own community or the wider Islamic community are very different from those of, for example, individuals who are right-wing militants in the United States. Whereas the latter typically appear to be marginalized individuals, among whom the rate of psychological disturbance and social awkwardness is quite high (Bakker and de Graaf, 2010), the former "justice seekers" are culled from largely middle-class, well-educated, and tightly knit families. Many are indeed exposed to radical beliefs, but for these to be internalized, they must resonate with their personal experience. It is for this reason that diasporas are so often fertile breeding grounds for radicalism, as the members of diasporas often find themselves marginalized economically and/or culturally in their host countries (McAllister and Schmid, 2011, p. 244).

Young and Male

It appears that while there is no evidence of psychopathic tendencies in recruits to illegal militias, there are some generic social and biopsychological processes that predispose people to become members of such militias. Criminally motivated violence is overwhelmingly the work of young unmarried men (Buvinic and Morrison, 1999). This is also true of those who join illegal militias. Recruits for violent extremist groups are generally male and young, and their gender, and attendant biological processes, often facilitate their engagement in such groups. The neural circuitry of young adult brains lights up different neural pathways than those in older adults, relying heavily on emotions and favoring sensory reward and immediacy and the excitement of action and of social bonding with peers over the potential future consequences of their actions. The emotional parts of our brains are particularly potent in those who are younger (Allard and Kensinger, 2014).

In addition, young men are flooded with testosterone, which makes them more likely to be risk-takers and eager to prove their masculinity (Steinberg, 2008). Depending on the environment, such characteristics can be positive or negative. As sociologists and criminologists know, there is a male-related age–crime curve that transcends all cultures, which is flat until about age ten and peaks at about eighteen. During this time, young men will often try to prove their status as tough and popular and, in some cases—depending on the environment and the opportunities available—will be aggressive and violent. The surge of testosterone leads to an impulse to prove oneself. For some this means being at their most aggressive and violent. Such levels of testosterone can also contribute to positive characteristics, which can be used for socially acceptable heroism, such as becoming firefighters, police officers, or soldiers.

The Heroic Quest

The search for significance is a fundamental human motivation (Kruglanski et al., 2013) and is particularly salient during adolescence. A "significance quest" model refers to the almost universal need for people to feel they make a difference, to be noteworthy, and to find one's purpose in life (Decety et al., 2018). Radicalism—the pursuit of fundamental political, economic, or social reforms—often provides a convenient track to such significance. It can enable young men to shape their individual identity and to find their place in a group (Dugas and Kruglanski, 2014). Such a quest for the heroic has always motivated young men to join violent movements and situations: the Christian Crusades, the Spanish Civil War, the IRA, Maoism, jihad groups, etc. By fighting, young men can quickly gain the status of heroes or, where such are valued, martyrs, particularly in contexts in which a young man's desire to gain individual significance is given little other opportunity to develop in a socially positive manner. In addition, abstract concepts such as justice and politics begin to have appeal as youths become busy building a new sense of identity. A match of perceived injustice and grievances allied with their identity search is a potent mix for recruiters to extreme groups (Hudson, 1999).

Studies conducted with members of the Sri Lankan terrorist organization the Liberation Tigers of Tamil Eelam found that feeling insignificant, or anger or shame, correlated with engaging in violent actions and supporting violent struggle against the Sinhalese majority (Webber et al., 2018). Martin McGuinness, a Catholic in a Protestant-dominated Northern Ireland and a major leader of the IRA, explained the reason for his allegiance during the years of oppression: he said that given what he and his friends in Londonderry/Derry (citizens of the city cannot agree on its name!) had endured at the hands of the British and the Ulster police, "I would have been ashamed not to join the IRA" (cited in Elmhirst, 2011).

For young men, joining a militia group can thus be about a sense of responsibility to address historical injustices or to provide for their families. In Nigeria, it was broad frustrations with the government that created initial community acceptance of Boko Haram, which took advantage of the deep grievances around government inadequacies and security abuses to gain acceptance in communities (Mercy Corps, 2016). Thus, many young men see violence as the only viable option left for them and their communities to regain any control over their lives. "Such young men convince themselves that they are righting epic wrongs, and many believe that their sacrifice (their 'martyrdom') is not only heroic but even chivalric" (Dickey, 2017).

The idea of adventure itself is enough to entice some young men to join militias. For example, the inherent risks or promise of exhilaration associated with terrorism may appeal primarily to individuals high in trait novelty-seeking or impulsivity (Victoroff, 2005). David Headley, who did much of the planning for the 2008 attacks in Mumbai, India, in which more than 160 people were killed, was not an observant Muslim. He apparently juggled multiple wives and girlfriends, was motivated by a passionate hatred of India, and found "enjoyment in playing the role of a jihadi James Bond, hanging out with Bollywood stars for cover while secretly planning one of the most spectacular and deadly terrorist assaults since Sept. 11, 2001" (Bergen, 2016). There is little doubt that young ISIS sympathizers, both male and female, are influenced by the glamor of images of a war with a cause, and by a "jihadi-cool subculture" including images of torture and executions of those who oppose the "caliphate." They are fascinated by the "cult of death" and by "heaven" and "life after death," and they talk about "five-star jihad" to describe the fun and excitement they are having fighting in Syria, rather than being "bored" in their home countries (Peresin, 2015).

Evidence given in an Irish court in 2000 at the a trial of a man named John McDonagh revealed that he had hung around a McDonald's in Dublin and recruited five young men for membership of a republican extremist group, Óglaigh na hÉireann (Young Men of Ireland), training camp. According to one fourteen-year-old, he had been told he would learn about Irish history, be shown guns, and be allowed to fire blanks. There was no evidence of any motivation for his joining other than a possible adventure (Wilson, 2000).

It appears that members of illegal militias who come from the United States and Western Europe in particular are often facing some sort of identity crisis and a desire for a personal sense of recognition that they cannot find at home. For those who find themselves alienated by the culture of their parents and do not feel they belong in the society within which they live, embracing a group that provides them with a sense of belonging and an opportunity to be a hero may be an attractive option.

Finding a Tribe

While it is often suggested that Western young men join illegal militias as the consequence of unsuccessful integration, this is simplistic and very much depends on the context. The fact is that most Muslims in, for example, France are somewhat socially integrated: in France, far more Muslims are enrolled in the police and security forces than are involved in jihad (Roy, 2017). Before they leave for jihad, many of the youth are often deeply immersed in youth culture, go to nightclubs, pick up girls, smoke and drink, and wear baseball caps and other fashionable youth streetwear. Nor do they live in a particularly religious environment—in fact many have an ambivalent relationship with the mosque, which they often attend only sporadically, and they do not often take part in proselytizing activities (Roy, 2007).

Adolescence and early adulthood are psychologically and hormonally confusing times. Adolescents are keen to "fit in" and belong, and a sense of isolation and vulnerability seems to be especially strong in young men in the world today. In almost every case, the processes by which a radical group in Europe is formed are nearly identical. Such recruitment is often facilitated by the lure of brothers and of friends, some of whom were made while a young man was in prison, who will encourage such membership (Roy, 2017).

Such a choice is usually made on the assumption of greater and deeper belonging to a group and a cause. Potential recruits are often unconsciously responding to the lure of another hormone—oxytocin. As we have seen in Chapter 3 of this volume, oxytocin increases a sense of belonging and of connectedness with a group and is heavily involved in rewarding the processes of group loyalty and belonging. It appears to be a relic from a mainly male ancestry. It has been shown that successful hunting increases testosterone, oxytocin, and cortisol in a subsistence population (Jaeggi et al., 2015). Given such biophysical rewards, it is no wonder that adolescents join gangs. However, although belonging to a group may strengthen their identity, it also makes them vulnerable to any form of extremism and to joining groups such as the Islamic State as part of a sort of "super-gang" (Dearden, 2016).

The rewards for group belonging are particularly desirable for those living in countries who are more collectivist in nature (see Chapter 7 of this volume). Based on surveys of thousands of people in fifteen Arab and other countries, researchers found that Muslims who have a more collectivistic mentality are more likely to support terrorist attacks against Americans or Europeans than those with more individualistic leanings (Dugas and Kruglanski, 2014).

Through the process of group membership, individuals establish kinship-like relationships within extremist organizations that open them up to sacrifices, such as acts of martyrdom, that are the price of group membership. "As such social bonds deepen, isolation from groups with competing values and the development of extreme beliefs facilitate interpersonal processes such as obedience, conformity, deindividuation, and dehumanization which, taken together, may set the stage for violence towards innocent individuals" (Decety et al., 2018). Individuals who become radicalized by such organizations usually withdraw from their previous social connections and from any groups whose values compete with membership of their new group, who often become their surrogate family. As individuals disconnect from formal and nonformal social groups to which they previously belonged and which were important to them, fewer connections to social groups with competing opinions and values result in a simpler adherence to extremist narratives, and this also decreases their openness to competing ideas. "Group dynamics, interpersonal factors, and micro-sociological factors interact reciprocally to create the conditions for hyper-altruism towards one's in-group as well as violent action directed at innocent out-group members" (Decety et al., 2018). As a consequence of such isolation from outside networks, terrorist groups often wield enormous influence over the behavior and values of their members.

Because of such alienating processes, group members' capacity for empathy—the emotion that enables people to better understand other people's intentions, feelings, and emotions and allows them to see the world from another's point of view—will also be affected. What seems to make many terrorists essentially different from others is their ability to "switch off" their sense of empathy in relation to their chosen beliefs and goals and toward those who do not share them. This may enable them to kill without remorse (Nehme, 2016).

The Need for Certainty

While extremist groups often provide a strong sense of belonging, assisted by the intoxication of oxytocin, they also often provide their adherents with certainty—that is, the conviction that they embody the truth, a conviction that is needed by some people more than others to stabilize their lives. Many researchers have found significant statistical relations between the need for closure and extremism (see Chapter 4 of this volume). This relationship was found regardless of where the researchers looked (e.g., Morocco, Spain, the Philippines, Palestine, Northern Ireland, Sri Lanka), although expressed differently through religious/cultural/political extremism (Dugas and Kruglanski, 2014).

Need for closure is a mindset that sees the world in sharp definition, with few shades of grey. Ideology paints a simplified ideal of the world people desire and of the world they want to eliminate. For ISIL, this means calling for young people to join in building the caliphate and to create a new, pure state uncorrupted by Western influences. For de Valera, the third president of Ireland, in 1943, it was building a romantic Ireland in which there would be happy "comely maidens" dancing at the crossroads of an independent rural state. For many in the United States today, it is "Make America Great Again." Such views are highly attractive to people who are seeking a clear-cut vision of life with which to identify. The elimination of ambiguity is particularly welcome to those who have a dislike of uncertainty and a high need for closure in their beliefs. Extremist views usually provide opportunities for such strict adherence to simplified versions of thoughts, beliefs, and world views (Bronner, 2016, p. 858; Horgan, 2014). For them, right and wrong are unambiguous, and their ideology provides them with a rationale for using violence as a means of re-establishing the balance between good and evil.

Memories are often destroyed in pursuit of such simplicity and hence the burning of books and the destruction of statues and buildings that portray differing beliefs to their own—the Bamiyan statues destroyed by the Taliban, certain translations of the Bible, the burning of mosques, etc. As Roy (2017) has noted, "wiping the slate clean" is a goal common to Mao Zedong's Red Guards, the Khmer Rouge, and ISIS fighters. One British jihadi wrote in a recruitment guide:

> When we descend on the streets of London, Paris and Washington . . . not only will we spill your blood, but we will also demolish your statues, erase your history and, most painfully, convert your children who will then go on to champion our name and curse their forefathers. (Roy, 2017)

Such simplicity of approach—such social purity—is not a need for most people, who will often compromise or nuance their moral values when this suits their interests and often hold contradictory beliefs. A tolerance for inconsistencies and ambiguities requires mental flexibility (i.e., the ability to shift between contradictory views), but such flexibility is difficult for those who crave certainty in a context that is often confusing or threatening.

The current world situation may constitute just such a context for many, as unprecedented waves of immigration dislocate millions of people, within a context of crumbling political orders. Amid all these uncertainties, adopting fundamentalist ideologies can help to satisfy cravings for certainty.

Interestingly, a study has shown that among jihadist militia who live in Muslim-majority countries, a high proportion are engineers, except in Saudi Arabia, where engineering skills are prized and engineers are far less likely to be underemployed (Gambetta and Hertog, 2016). The authors of the study propose two possible explanations: unmet professional expectations and personality types. The latter includes a desire to draw rigid boundaries between insiders and outsiders and a need for cognitive closure, which traits, they argue, based on survey data, are stronger among engineers and weaker among humanities and social science graduates.

Sexual Rewards

An important but often overlooked factor in the recruitment for illegal militias in the Middle East is the use of sexual rewards as an attraction for men. Abu Bakr al-Baghdadi, the self-declared caliph of ISIS, ordered that a marriage grant be given to all members of ISIL who wanted to enter matrimony, which included housing and a sum of $1,200. So many were the ISIL fighters who were unmarried and wanted a wife that they opened a "marriage bureau" for women who wanted to wed the group's fighters in Syria and Iraq. Such offerings are very attractive to testosterone-filled young men, many of whom have lived in societies or communities where premarital sex is forbidden and who had no obvious way of earning enough to enter into a normal marriage. Such offerings double the sexual rewards available for fighting: the provision of current sexual partners along with the promise that should they die in battle or in a suicide attack, they will attain the status of martyrs, whose ultimate reward is marrying beautiful virgins on entry into paradise.

Thus, ISIS has turned the strategic use of sexual favors into a well-oiled machine.

> Young, often sexually frustrated men are promised sexual Shangri-La for their bravery: there are brides eager to marry them, their rape of non-believers is legitimized, sexual slaves can be purchased (through ISIL mediation) and fatwas are issued proclaiming a "sexual jihad," forcing girls to be married to militants. (Kruglanski, Bélanger, and Gunaratna, 2019, p. 54)

Why Do Women Join Illegal Militias?

Women's participation in violent extremism is nothing new. Research has estimated that currently women represent, on average, between 10 and 15 percent of extremist groups' membership (Lunz and Dier, 2019). They have been active participants in 60 percent of armed rebel groups over the past decades. In Algeria in the 1950s, they deployed bombs in the cities. In the 1970s and 1980s, many women played prominent roles in the liberation movements in Latin America and in European terrorist networks. In 1983, the Liberation Tigers of Tamil Eelam founded a special section for women who were trained for combat: estimates vary, but they are believed to have constituted from 15 percent to 33 percent of the core battle strength. In Colombia, women represented nearly 40 percent of FARC. The Syrian Kurdish resistance has made a point of including women among its fighters, and its all-women unit (YPJ) claims to have more than more than 20,000 members. Women have also been involved as violent extremists in the Shining Path group in Peru, in Northern Ireland, in Turkey through the Kurdistan Workers Party, and in the Philippines through Abu Sayyaf (Agara, 2015, p. 116; Banks, 2019) and in acts of terror in insurgencies and uprisings in Pakistan, India, Sri Lanka, Chechnya, Afghanistan, Palestine, Syria, Iraq, Yemen, and Kenya (Gentry and Sjoberg, 2016, p. 149; Weinberg and Eubank, 2011, pp. 23–25). In Nigeria, female members of Boko Haram have been so effective in killing more than 1,200 people between 2014 and 2018 that women now comprise close to two-thirds of the group's suicide attackers ("Why Boko Haram Uses Female Suicide-Bombers," 2017).

In Europe, women constituted 26 percent of those arrested on terrorism charges in 2016, up from 18 percent the previous year (Bigio and Turkington,

2019). The number of women—mostly Muslim, but not all—from the West who joined ISIS is estimated to represent 10 percent of all ISIS's Western foreign fighters (Sherwood et al., 2014). The number of women implicated in terrorism-related crimes is growing. In 2017, the Global Extremism Monitor registered 100 distinct suicide attacks conducted by 181 female militants, 11 percent of all incidents that year (Tony Blair Institute for Global Change, 2018).

Why Do Women Join?

For some women, joining a group as an active militant is not voluntary: for example, in Nigeria, Boko Haram uses many of the women it has kidnapped as suicide bombers, who have no choice in whether or not they take up militant roles ("Why Boko Haram Uses Female Suicide-Bombers," 2017). Others choose voluntarily to join such groups for varied reasons—to right injustice, to increase their power as women, or to seek excitement and romance. Women in the Tamil Tigers often said they joined because of the treatment of their fellow Hindus under the Sinhalese government. Others joined to avenge family members who had been killed by enemy combatants (Wall and Choksi, 2018). Still others said they joined because of rapes committed by the Indian peacekeeping force (Press Trust of India, 2014). For others, joining the militia was their first taste of freedom, and they saw it as a chance to fight for equality by taking on traditionally masculine roles (Alison, 2003). For many Kurdish women, their voluntary recruitment for military roles was also a fight for women's rights, and the war was a fight against patriarchy (Lazarus, 2019).

While many Islamic societies were actively opposed to the use of women soldiers, that changed as the men began to understand how useful women could be to their causes. In August 2001, the Saudi High Council officially authorized women to participate in terrorist attacks in the name of jihad (Davis, 2006). Subsequently, Hamas's spiritual leader, Sheikh Yassin, condoned the employment of women as suicide bombers and inducements were offered—for example, women would be reunited with their husbands in paradise as a reward for their commitment or with an arranged marriage to a Hamas member if they were unmarried when alive (Banks, 2019; Margolin, 2016, pp. 919–920). Today there are few limits on the recruitment of women for jihadi war.

Western women are proactively lured by internet ads posted by ISIS/ISIL pimps, both male and female, which appeal to their desire to be part of something larger than themselves, including the appeal of "sisterhood," a desire to be part of the state-building effort of ISIS, or to be part of something "bigger and divine" (Grierson, 2019). Many are enticed by the promise of a new life with strong, heroic, and devout men who they believe will look after them and protect them. "It's an idea, it's like movies" (Paton Walsh et al., 2017). ISIS female recruits are also promised a free house, equipped with top-of-the-line appliances, and all expenses paid to convince them that they will be financially secure and will not miss out on anything in life.

For some women, the result is indeed a "proper" romance and an Islamic marriage, and they are happy to stay in the Middle East with their husband and children. However, forced inseminations and pregnancies are often officially endorsed to help secure the next generation of jihadis. In addition, "holy war brides" are often required to take turns with the militia members for sexual relations, with no say in the matter, due to the idea of temporary marriages, which is legally enshrined in Islamic religious law. If a woman is Western and blonde, she may be taken on for sex trafficking and find herself sold into the harems of Saudi Arabia, Brunei, or the Gulf States (McFadyen and Pallenberg, 2016). Such practices have long been an attraction for male militias of all kinds. The Vikings' freedom to "rape and pillage" has unfortunately been the way of many, if not all, wars, as records from Japan, Serbia, Pakistan, Peru, Bosnia, Rwanda, Congo, Iraq, etc. can testify (Benedict, 2008). Rape has become an established recruiting tool to lure men from deeply conservative Muslim societies, where casual sex is taboo and dating is forbidden (Callimachi, 2015).

Western women who become involved with nonstate armed organizations come from a range of backgrounds. In terms of educational background, most scholars agree that women fighters are at least as educated as their peers outside their group (Eggert, 2018). Many of these women believe that they are taking part in a humanitarian mission toward other Muslims, and this is used by ISIS recruiters to boost their aspirations to live and practice their religion in a more congenial environment (Peresin, 2015). For other women, it is a chance to prove themselves: ISIL's English and French propaganda materials sought to portray messages of female empowerment, geared specifically toward Western women whom they hoped to entice to travel to the conflict zone.

Conclusion

The involvement of young men, and an increasing number of young women, in violent extremism is often aided by a perfect storm of their youthful hormonal tendencies, allied with a particular genetic make-up, and an environment (at home or abroad) that is seen as unjust or excluding. Motivations will differ; for example, joining such militias is often a material or psychological survival necessity, particularly for young men, in some conflict contexts. In the West, however, it is often those whose idealistic or responsibility capacities are not being utilized and who are offered a chance to engage in actions that offer brotherhood (and increasingly sisterhood) and meaning who are easy targets for recruitment to fundamentalist and violent causes. It is important to note that contexts, whether at home or abroad, that involve political and social identity inequalities are like tinderboxes ready to explode when triggered by leaders who offer violent ways to address these inequalities (see Chapter 6 of this volume).

6

Follow the Leader

My president needs bravado . . . somebody who is big and loud,
strong and powerful.
> —Victoria Wilen (quoted in "Election 2016," 2016)

War remains primarily an instrument of politics in the hands of
willful leaders.
> —Carnegie Corporation of New York (1997)

Introduction

- James Warren Jones was an American cult leader of a commune at
  Jonestown, Guyana. Under his orders, 918 commune members committed suicide, having previously killed 304 of their children by cyanide-
  poisoned Flavor Aid.
- Pol Pot, the Cambodian Khmer Rouge leader, was responsible for killing
  between 1.2 million and 2.8 million of his own people.
- Joseph Stalin was responsible for ordering the execution of over a million people and sending millions more to work as slaves and perish in
  the Gulag.
- Under Adolf Hitler's regime, over 6 million Jews and 11 million others
  were tortured and murdered.

How was—and is—it possible that so many apparently ordinary, decent
people end up, often voluntarily, supporting brutal and murderous leaders?

The quality of leaders is critical to both war-making and peacebuilding.
The disposition and the skills of leaders can make the difference between
conflicts that are solved through processes of politics, law, or social and economic development and those that proceed more violently (Horowitz, Stam,
and Ellis, 2016). Unfortunately, it appears that it is often far easier for groups
to choose a leader to make war rather than peace. Warlords and divisive

Our Brains at War. Mari Fitzduff, Oxford University Press (2021). © Oxford University Press.
DOI: 10.1093/oso/9780197512654.003.0007

politicians seem to abound, while peacelords and inclusive politicians—leaders who are trusted by their own group but also adept at connecting across identity boundaries so as to help ensure peaceful societies or to craft peace processes—are notoriously difficult to find (Peake and Fitzduff, 2004). Why is this so?

Choosing Our Leaders

Choosing and following leaders is part of the human process by which we organize our groups, our societies, and our nations—sometimes for the better but sometimes for the worse. Our mode of choosing our leaders is often a mismatch between characteristics that used to be useful in our ancestors' lives and what might be useful for our societal and global needs today. Due to our emotional heritage, we often make automatic judgments regarding a person's leadership suitability without thinking deeply about their actual skills (Shondrick and Lord, 2010). It appears that our choices of leaders are often more instinctual than rational and are influenced not only by our social networks but also by our genetics, our brain structures, and hormones such as adrenaline, norepinephrine, and cortisol, which inform our response to messages from leaders, particularly those who message uncertainties or fear.

From early childhood we have an instinctual sense about who we think would make a good leader, well before mature rationality comes in to play. One study has found that children as young as five years old can pick the winners of political elections based only on photos of the faces of the candidates (Antonakis and Dalgas, 2009). As adults, many of us often make inferences on leadership competence in a fraction of a second (Tskhay, Zoo, and Rule, 2014) using non-conscious processing and non-verbal and unexamined cues to assist our decisions.

When asked to identify the reasons why they prefer a particular candidate, people often offer unclear or seeming illogical answers to justify their choices. This supremacy of emotions in choosing our leaders is particularly relevant in "weak psychological situations" such as crises, conflicts, or situations characterized by uncertainty (Mischel, 1973)—all factors that are inherently present in most conflict contexts and in the world today. The research shows that people's implicit leadership theories change to favor more forceful leaders when they feel anxious and insecure. Thus when we are told that we are being threatened by other countries, by terror attacks, or by influxes of immigrants, a leader taps into our amygdala fears, which often overwhelm the cortex thinking that is needed for us to rationally choose the leader that is needed for today's complex and changing situations. An autocratic leader need only instill uncertainty to gather support: several studies show that the limbic system in the brain can treat uncertainty as even more threatening and dangerous than actual threats (Rock, 2016). Thus, *fear often chooses our leaders for us.*

So, why are our instincts for choosing particular leaders so powerful? It has been suggested that our ability to detect leadership may have developed as a survival mechanism in our history. Because humans evolved as primarily a group-living species (Dunbar, 2004), leadership processes were specifically designed to solve many challenges that needed solving to ensure the successful survival of the group. It appears that the requirements for leaders evolved in response to long-term environmental factors, especially the availability of food (Wrangham and Peterson, 1996). Such environmental factors have become ingrained in our brains and bodies and initiate automatic responses that occur beyond our conscious control (Jost et al., 2014). Thus, many factors in leadership choices are biologically based and have long been programmed into our psyches as part of hierarchal structures that fostered our survival and safety many thousands of years ago (Fowler and Schreiber, 2008).

Robert Lord and his colleagues (Lord, Foti, and De Vader, 1984; Lord and Maher, 1991) have introduced the concept of implicit leadership theory to explain such leadership choices. Implicit leadership theory suggests that group members have implicit expectations and assumptions about the personal characteristics, traits, and qualities that are inherent in a leader. Many studies have shown that facial and bodily appearances and gestures matter a lot in the people we select as leaders. People infer leadership traits from a leader's body language during speeches and not necessarily from the content of such speeches (Koppensteiner and Grammer, 2010; Stewart, Waller, and Schubert, 2009), Such theories can help explain why, even in today's world, leadership suitability is often contingent on the match between facial cues indicating, for example, dominance and competence and perceived follower needs (Van Vugt and Grabo, 2015).

It seems our prime criterion for leaders is often apparent strength. Height is seen as an indicator of strength (Van Vugt, Hogan, and Kaiser, 2008), as are mouth width (Re and Rule, 2016) and lower pitched voice (Klofstad, Anderson, and Nowicki, 2015). Nonverbal body language signals (Reh, Van

Quaquebeke, and Giessner, 2017) as well as general physical indices such as energy level and health are also often correlated with leadership (Spisak et al., 2014). Apparently, facial displays and physical gestures better predict followers' responses during a presidential debate than the candidates' message, and these displays can alter viewers' emotional state (Bucy, 2000; Shah, Hanna, and Bucy, 2015). Thus, based on the presence (or absence) of such body signals, researchers can now explain—even predict and (to a certain degree) control—who wins most democratic elections, regardless of the so-called campaign issues (Dumitrescu, Gidengil, and Stolle, 2015).

People tend to follow figures who are sensed as strong and resolute, particularly when threatened by war (McCann, 1992) or when experiencing crisis (Pillai, 1996). For example, when people were asked to choose a president assuming the country was at war, more people voted for a candidate whose face was perceived as more masculine (Laustsen and Petersen, 2015). However, they prefer leaders with more trustworthy faces in peacetime (Little et al., 2012). In addition, leaders with older-looking faces are preferred in traditionally more stable societies, whereas younger-looking leaders are preferred for apparently new challenges (Van Vugt and Grabo, 2015).

Researchers have discovered that voters rate speakers with low-pitched voices as higher for attractiveness, leadership potential, honesty, intelligence, and dominance (Tigue et al., 2011). They thus suggest that female politicians' chances of success are rated as higher if they learn to modulate their voices downwards on the hustings!

Who is perceived as a good leader is also influenced by a leader's neuro-endocrine system (e.g., testosterone, cortisol, and oxytocin), which regulates hormone levels. These hormones are responsible for many of the traits associated with either strong or weak leadership, such as the ability to read people, levels of dominance, resilience, and anxiety (Davis and Mehta, 2015). Another factor that suggests that women leaders may have a harder climb than men is the fact that researchers have found that the most effective leaders have high levels of testosterone, which is associated with competitive behavior and sensitivity to status. They also have lower levels of cortisol—the hormone that comes into play in highly pressurized situations—and thus are better able to adapt in high-pressure situations, where raised cortisol levels and associated anxiety could diminish their leadership skills (Adams, 2015; Davis and Mehta, 2015).

Such instinctual choices often persist through the actual performance of leadership positions. It appears that having chosen their leaders, followers also tolerate "bad leaders" for non-cognitive reasons; often simply because they are "tall dark, and handsome" (Bridgeman, 2003, p. 84).

Once in power, it is easy for our leaders to become addicted to power. The primary neurochemical involved in the chemical rewarding of power is do-pamine, which is the chemical transmitter responsible for producing a sense of pleasure. It seems that power activates the dopamine reward circuitry in the brain and thus creates an addictive "high" that many in power will seek to maintain. "When withheld, power —like any highly addictive agent — produces cravings at the cellular level that generate strong behavioural op-position to giving it up" (Al-Rodham, 2014). Hence, many leaders, even in supposedly democratic countries, are reluctant to resign.

Interestingly, genetic traits do not seem to disproportionally affect leader-ship traits. Arvey et al. (2006) have done extensive work using twins to show that perhaps only 30 percent of the variance in leaders can be accounted for by genetics, while non-shared (or non-common) environmental factors accounted for the remaining variance. De Neve et al. (2013), using twin studies, have estimated the genetic heritability of leadership roles at 24 per-cent. The results show that what determines whether an individual occupies a leadership position is a complex product of genetic and environmental influences, which includes a particular role for a genotype, called rs4950 which appears to be associated with the passing of leadership ability down through generations (De Neve et al., 2013).

A "toxic" leader is one who abuses the leader–follower relationship by leaving the group or organization in a worse condition than they found it in (Whicker, 1996). It seems that to be successful, such toxic leaders need an environment where they can thrive. Yapp (2016) suggests that four elem-ents contribute to a conducive environment for toxic leaders: instability, perceived threat, questionable values and standards, and an absence of gov-ernance. Toxic leaders will take advantage of—and seek to create—these types of environments. Padilla, Hogan, and Kaiser (2007) have written about the "toxic triangle" of destructive leaders, susceptible followers, and con-ducive environments. It seems that charismatic and egotistical leaders take their greatest hold among followers who "lack self-assurance or who share the leader's ambition and selfishness. They are particularly vulnerable to such leaders in situations marked by instability, individualism, or lack of account-ability" (Rock, 2016). Thus, to succumb to, for example, Hitler's charisma, Laurence Rees (quoted in Romano, 2013) argues that "it helped immensely to be hungry or humiliated by the First World War and Versailles, to be unemployed or feel betrayed by democracy, to be eager to put the blame on someone else."

Hitler's charismatic persuasiveness was also deeply connected with his capacity to connect emotionally with his audience. According to Romano (2013), he rooted his hatreds in "an emotionality that was given such free rein as to appear out of control. The ability to feel events emotionally and to demonstrate that emotion to others was a crucial part of his charismatic appeal." Another observer reflected that Hitler's persuasive impact came from his ability to strategically express emotions—he would "tear open his heart"—and these emotions affected his followers to the point that they would "stop thinking critically and just emote" (Grant, 2014). It appears that when a leader gives an inspiring speech filled with emotion, the audience are less likely to scrutinize the message and to remember the content.

Interestingly, the important effect of emotional body language was recognized early by Hitler, who spent years studying it. According to the historian Roger Moorhouse (quoted in Grant, 2014), practicing his hand gestures and analyzing images of his movements allowed him to become "an absolutely spellbinding public speaker." Apparently leaders who master the power of their—and our—emotions can rob us of our capacity to think too deeply. According to Volkan (2004), divisive leaders often capitalize on the influence of chosen traumas (see Chapter 3 of this volume) within a group. They attempt to reawaken and emphasize collective memories, emotions, and prejudices to solidify their power and ideals. Through such memories, manipulative leaders can encourage an aggressive feeling for the ideals of nationalism, tribalism, and ethnocentrism.

Such was the power of the Serbian leader Slobodan Milosevic. As a fairly inconsequential Serb Communist leader, in 1997, he seized on the issue of Kosovo and the perceived freedoms that were permitted to the 90-percent Albanian majority in the province that many Serbs regarded as the ancient "heartland" of their collective traumatized memory. As tensions were rising over this situation, Milosevic told the Serbs in Kosovo that "nobody shall beat you"—a phrase that resonated around the country (Crawshaw, 1998). Such leadership became the cause of the death of an estimated 100,000 people, including in July 1995 in the town of Srebrenica, when Bosnian Serb forces killed as many as 8,000 Bosnian men and boys. It was the largest massacre in Europe since the Holocaust.

Followership

Why do people so easily follow both good and bad leaders? It appears that hierarchies form spontaneously in human groups and that humans have an in-built bias to follow leaders (Van Vugt et al., 2008) and punish deviants (O'Gorman, Henrich, and Van Vugt, 2008). Obedience studies show how easy it is for us to do harm to others. In an infamous experiment, when Milgram (1963) ordered his subjects to hurt individuals with ever-increasing intensity, even when it meant causing apparently substantial pain to others, they obeyed him.

Low self-esteem, locus of control, and self-efficacy are linked to a vulnerability to destructive leadership (e.g., Luthans, Peterson, and Ibrayeva, 1998). Individuals with low self-esteem often wish to be someone more desirable, which prompts them to identify with charismatic leaders (Hoffer, 1951; Shamir, Arthur, and House, 1994). When followers link leaders with salient aspects of their own self-concept, emotional attachments form between them (Lord and Brown, 2003). The closer the leader is to the follower's self-concept, the stronger the bond and the greater the motivation to follow (Belasen, 2015, p. 187). Behaving in ways that are consistent with the leader's vision and the follower's self-concept boosts self-esteem and self-efficacy (Shamir, House, and Arthur, 1993; Weierter, 1997). Followers with world views that are similar to those of a destructive leader are more likely to join their cause (Raffy, 2004). Followers' values are also relevant; that is, individuals who endorse unsocialized values such as greed and selfishness are more likely to follow destructive leaders and engage in destructive behavior (Hogan, 2006). Undersocialized followers who are ambitious are more likely to engage in destructive acts, especially if they are permitted or encouraged by a leader (McClelland, 1975).

Followers often passively allow bad leaders to assume power because their unmet needs make them vulnerable to such leaders, and they support such leaders because they want to promote themselves in an enterprise that is matched with their own needs (Padilla et al., 2007). Transference—a situation where the feelings, desires, and expectations of a person in relation to someone in their past are redirected and applied to another person—is often the emotional glue that binds people to a leader. Transferences makes their leaders seem smarter and more charismatic than they are: followers tend to give that person the benefit of the doubt and take on more risk at their request than they otherwise would (Maccoby, 2004). Interestingly, people are often most swayed by leaders on whom they have little information, which means they can fill the gaps by projecting their own needs and wishes onto the leader.

We also have a desire to imitate higher-status individuals (Brody and Stoneman, 1985). Our choice of apparently strong leaders is assisted by what is called "referent power," coined by Thorndike in 1920, which is a follower's willingness to devote themselves to a particular leader because of that person's known celebrity or other status (Dacko, 2008, p. 248). A related concept is the "positive attribution error": when we see the actions of another person, we believe that it reflects their personality rather than the situation they might be in (L. Ross, 1977). Allied to this is a cognitive bias called the "halo effect," whereby an observer's overall impression of the success of a person in one sphere will be taken to mean that they will be successful in another (L. Ross, 1977). Leaders are often chosen from the military—for example, in Israel—for such reasons. It has also been suggested that the selection of President Trump in the United States was facilitated by the halo effect of his apparent ruthlessness in dealing with participants on the *Apprentice* TV show.

Inspiring leaders can make followers feel absolved of the responsibility to do anything hard. People with an external locus of control, who believe that outcomes are determined by external factors, versus those with an internal locus of control, who believe that one's own efforts determine one's fate (Rotter, 1966), are easier to manipulate and are attracted to others who seem powerful and willing to care for them (Padilla et al., 2007). According to Kohlberg, Levine, and Hewer (1983), it appears that psychologically immature individuals are more likely to conform to authority and to participate in destructive acts. Some research suggests that such morally immature individuals include between 60 and 75 percent of Western adults (Cook-Greuter, 1999).

Unfortunately, followers can be very easily deceived—and such deception appears to be second nature to many leaders. It usually involves deliberately underselling the costs and overselling the benefits for their followers of what they are proposing—as well as overselling their own contribution and underselling the benefits that they personally receive (White, 2017).

However, while it is the followers' psychological qualities that render them susceptible to the force of charismatic leaders (Ulman and Apse, 1983), the relationship between the leader and the followers is often complex and changeable. Schiffer (1973) has observed that all leaders, especially charismatic leaders, are at heart the creation of their followers within a particular context. As Post (2004, p. 262) has said, "one cannot understand the destructive charismatic leadership of Osama Bin Laden without addressing the psychology of the alienated, despairing Islamic youth to whom he appeals." In situations where people have felt attacked:

> feelings of humiliation may lead to rage, that may be turned inwards, as in the case of depression and apathy. However, this rage may also turn outwards and express itself in violence, even in mass violence, in case leaders are around who forge narratives of humiliation that feed on the feelings of humiliation among the masses. (Lindner, 2006, p. 141)

As previously noted, the identification of a leader appears, to some great extent, a nonconscious, System 1 decision, as per Kahneman's work (2011) described in Chapter 2 of this volume. Thus we instinctively (although often unconsciously) follow our impressions and feelings in choosing our leaders. System 2 thinking is slower, examines facts, and applies cost–benefit analyses to our choices. The latter process appears to matter a lot less for most of us in choosing leaders. In listening to a political candidate, we often quickly conclude that the person is or is not fit for office without a great deal of deliberative thought about their qualifications.

Unfortunately, many leaders use such feelings to foment wars. To achieve power, they often involve themselves in "ethnic outbidding" and encourage or command atrocities to be committed by their followers. Given the tendencies toward followership, it can be seen how easily identity groups of a racial, religious, social, or ethnic nature can be grist to the mill of most of our wars around the world today and how leaders can easily utilize almost any categorization for their own purposes.

Societal differences serve as ever-ready fodder for leaders and would-be leaders. Gathering out-group bias is perhaps the most common strategy that leaders use to persuade followers to work together and to bring them to or keep them in power. While this has always been part of a national strategy for war, today's context, with its increasingly diverse societies, supplies leaders with an ever-increasing number of supposed out-groups within national borders that provide a perfect basis for appealing to voters by signaling where they can direct their anger. By insulting out-groups, leaders can help their own groups to "achieve high self-esteem and increase their perception of power, to create distance with people they detest, to stress their advantages in comparison with others, to blame others for their own inappropriate actions, and to increase legitimacy of their views and positions" (Korostelina, 2014, p. 154). These followers love the fact that, on their behalf, leaders will often blame and insult those they feel (or are told) are the ones responsible for their economic and social bad luck.

As well as wanting to see strength on the part of their leaders, voters prefer simple messages: they like their leaders to give them simple slogans, rather than complex information about problems or strategies to address the challenges. Such simple phrases and viewpoints, which may offer little in the way of substance but are evocative in terms of feelings, are often very successful in building up a following. People also like their leaders to be un-compromising and prefer them to speak with certitude about issues they are concerned about—irrespective of the substance of their arguments. German listeners loved the fact that Hitler spoke with "conviction" and "absolute cer-tainty" (Romano, 2013). Hitler's own thinking revealed an intolerance of ambiguity and a high need for structure and cognitive closure that is charac-teristic of authoritarians (Suedfeld and Schaller, 2002). Leaders who express uncertainty and espouse consultation often make people feel uneasy. Hence the many objections to US President Obama as "weak" because of the time and care he took to consult with others on major decisions.

People often feel profoundly uncomfortable with the idea of uncertainty and with associated nuances that worry them and make them anxious. Strange as it may seem, studies have shown that candidates may actually vote for people with whom they disagree but who are supported by ideologies (and leaders) that are most likely to satisfy their current psychological needs and motives. These usually include their needs for order, structure, closure, and the avoidance of uncertainty or threat (Kakkar and Sivanathan, 2017; Lipman-Blumen, 2006).

It appears that our attachment to democracy is weak, and even weaker in contexts that are uncertain and fearful. Even in developed countries with an apparently strong democracy, people are prepared to abandon many dem-ocratic principles (Lipman-Blumen, 2007). In the United States, it seems that when the need for strengthening security appears to conflict with the values of freedom and human rights, the need for security prevails (G. Ross, 2011). The 2011 US-based World Values Survey (2011) found that 34 per-cent of US Americans approved of "having a strong leader who doesn't have to bother with Congress or elections," with the figure rising to 42 percent among those with no education beyond high school. Almost one in three US citizens would prefer a dictator to democracy. This is particularly true in people with a disposition toward authoritarianism, who often demonstrate a greater readiness to follow and obey strong leaders. While such authoritarian tendencies are not a stable personality trait, they can easily be activated when someone's social or economic context becomes threatening to the individual or group.

It is important to remember, however, that while it appears to be extraordinarily easy for leaders to frame conflicts divisively, it is not just the leader who elicits such conflicts. Leaders are assisted by the fact that people often already have negative predispositions against rivals/out-groups because of historical or current prejudices or grievances. Such predispositions may prompt followers to respond emotionally to divisive stimuli such as political rhetoric, events, and actions taken by leaders. An experimental study that presented participants with a speech from a fabricated congressional candidate proposing anti-Muslim policies (religious markers on identification cards, etc.) found that individuals with a pre-existing dislike for Muslims were emotionally moved by the speech, which prompted support for the exclusion policies. Conversely, individuals not having anti-Muslim attitudes were turned off by the speech and rejected the policies (Grillo, 2017). Thus, followers with dispositions to authoritarianism are permitted by a divisive leader to allow their prejudices to come to the surface. The leader enables them to feel comfortable with and express their prejudices and align their surfacing views with those of the leader.

It can be difficult for followers to reverse their first impressions of a leader, as this would require them to disentangle themselves from what are often automatic processes and to actively consider new pieces of information (Mann and Ferguson, 2015). The reality is that once people have emotionally adopted a leader, even new negative information about that leader can often lead them to intensify rather than lessen their support for him, her, or them (but mostly him).

Obviously, the qualities people seek in a leader will vary across cultures. For example, comparative studies (Den Hartog et al., 1999; Gerstner and Day, 1994; Hofstede et al., 2010) have shown that followers in various cultures have different "leadership schemas" arising from exposure to different historical cultures, textbooks, novels, movies, and other channels of socialization (Popper, 2012; also see Chapter 7 of this volume).

"Good" Leadership—The Holy Grail

What constitutes "good" leadership or "bad" leadership often depends on context and is often defined, of course, by the victors who write the history of wars. Thus those who would perhaps be identified as "terrorists" today are often those lauded as leaders at a later stage in their lives. Yesterday's warlords and militia commanders are often today's civic leaders.

So what is particular about the "good" leadership that peacebuilders would usually see as desirable in the peacebuilding work of today's increasingly diverse world? Here it may be useful to note the distinction between what Burns (1978) and Judge and Piccolo (2004) have termed "transformational" and "transactional" leadership.

In most conflict situations, leaders and followers are locked into what is called a "transactional" contract: leaders will usually act with a high degree of awareness about what their followers want, and their leadership is based on their ability to deliver this. Where they think it necessary, they will often deepen the differences between their group and the perceived enemies and appeal to emotions of their followers such as confusion, insecurity, fear, and hatred. Leaders serving only themselves, their party, and/or their identity group are the norm in many of the conflicts that have happened since the end of the Cold War. Those who exercise power, as Milosevic did, by promoting group against group—by promising a win/lose goal to the conflict—are often the main energizer of violence.

Transformational leaders, on the other hand, appeal to the higher motivations of their followers—that is, their ability to see beyond the group's immediate self-interest and to mobilize parties in a conflict to seek a greater common good for all in the conflict context. Transformational leaders involved in peacebuilding will communicate their inclusive beliefs in a way that will encourage their followers to expand their circle of concern from their own narrow concern to a wider societal one in which the views and needs of all within a community or society or nation or region—or, ultimately, the world—are taken into account.

The neurological correlates with transformational leaders have been recorded in many studies. One study, which involved a two-step, neural variable reduction and selection process, was claimed to be 92.5 percent accurate in its classification of both civilian and military leaders on the basis of their electroencephalogram trace. Focusing on transformational leadership, the findings point to the role of various frontal brain areas, including those associated with executive functions (such as planning and foresight), the effective handling of emotions (managing one's own and others'), and the right frontal region, largely responsible for adding meaning and nuance to verbal communication (Balthazard et al., 2012).

Research has also shown that the right brains of leaders who were willing to build a social vision (emphasis on social responsibility, altruism, stakeholders' authorization) could be identified, and they were almost the same as those of leaders who were described by, for example, organizational employees as incentive/charismatic leaders (Waldman, Balthazard, and Peterson, 2011).

A prime example of transformational leadership was the donning by Nelson Mandela in 1995 of the jersey of the predominantly white South Africa team in front of a mostly white and Afrikaner crowd at the Rugby World Cup final. Through this act, the future of South Africa was changed: "When the final whistle blew this country changed for ever. It's incomprehensible" (South Africa captain Francois Pienaar, quoted in D. Smith, 2013). There have been a few other such leaders (e.g., Martin Luther King, Mahatma Gandhi), who sought an inclusive approach to their particular conflicts and exercised their leadership to that end.

Unfortunately, transformation leaders can be difficult to find in the peacebuilding context. A 2004 study of leadership, which this author supervised, studied the apparently developing peace processes in Kosovo, Sierra Leone, and Afghanistan, showing that few of the traditional leaders had actually managed to transcend the essentially transactionalist nature of their relationship with their followers. Most of them exercised what is called "chameleonic leadership"—an inconstant leadership that shifted according to the opinions of others, the funds available from donors, and the climate in which the conflict operated. Local leaders were mostly just pretending to be inclusive in their leadership policies, while secretly favoring their own tribe or people. There seemed little likelihood that they would continue such an inclusive, transformational approach when the international funding that was assisting the development of such policies ended (Peake, Gormley, and Fitzduff, 2004).

Conclusion

As the complexity of the modern state increases, leadership failure may become more common, and cooperation between leaders and followers more difficult to sustain. Today some scholars observe that we are faced with a leadership crisis, as many leaders appear to hold power for no understandable reason other than their followers' fear. Many of today's researchers argue that we can explain much of current leadership behavior in terms of the mismatch between our old brains and the new context in which we function (Van Vugt and Ahuja, 2010). While economic, communications, and environmental interdependency is increasing and globalizing throughout the world, many of our old-style leaders are still prevailing, often having been chosen on the basis of what are now possibly outdated notions of leadership. This theory is called the mismatch hypothesis, and it suggests that very often the cues we use to seek leadership are based on past needs rather than present-day contexts in which groups are considerably larger and often significantly more diverse and where weapons for survival depend on nuclear buttons and drone dexterity much more than physical strength. This leads some evolutionary psychologists to conclude that "our modern skulls house a Stone Age mind" (Tooby and Cosmides, 1990): the leaders that suited our ancestors and their survival may not suit the human race today.

7

Accultured Norms

When you have a diverse group of people from different cultures,
you get not just different beliefs about the world, but different ways
of perceiving it and reasoning about it, each with its own strengths
and weaknesses.

—R. E. Nisbett (cited in "How Culture Colors," 2000)

Introduction

It had seemed like a good idea—bringing Israeli and Palestinian journalists
to Boston for some joint training in reporting for their various media. I had
been asked to facilitate some intergroup dialogue on the afternoon of the first
day of the course. I duly arrived at the studios to find (as I had half expected,
being familiar with such groups) that hostilities had already emerged between the groups, who had met for the first time that morning. Grim faces
abounded.

The conflict seemed simple to the Israelis. Here they all were, having
agreed to spend a week training together, and the Palestinians had refused to
have a group photo taken with them. The Israelis could not understand this—
and indeed some felt insulted at the Palestinians' refusal. What they had not
understood was something that social psychology, and increasingly social
neuroscience, could demonstrate: that while Israelis, akin to Westerners in
many of their characteristics, tend to view themselves as independent entities, the Palestinians tend to construe themselves in a manner that is more
sensitive to their context and to existing group relationships. The Israelis felt
that such a joint photo would only send a message to their families and communities about how liberal they as people were. What slowly emerged during
the course of the discussion was that the Palestinians were concerned that a
group photo with Israelis would send the wrong message to their communities back in Israel, the West Bank, and Gaza. Their fear was related to how

Our Brains at War. Mari Fitzduff, Oxford University Press (2021). © Oxford University Press.
DOI: 10.1093/oso/9780197512654.003.0008

they might be seen as fraternizing with the enemy back home in a context where intragroup relationships were often a more critical factor than independence of thought.

The Importance of Understanding Culture

"Culture" has been defined in many, many ways (Spencer-Oatey, 2012). For the purpose of this chapter I have defined it as the collective feeling, thinking, and behavior of a group of people that distinguishes interactions within the group, and between it and other people and groups, on norms that are relevant to peacebuilding work. Without understanding such differences, peacebuilding work, even with the best of motivations, can be fraught with challenges. The price for such misunderstanding can be high. Having "liberated" Iraq in 2003, it was 2007 before the US military set up the Center for Advanced Operational Culture Learning and a predeployment course to train its soldiers on how to work sensitively with the local populations ("Coaching US Troops," 2007). The program included Arab culture, Islamic etiquette, gender issues, and language course requirements. As Barack Salmoni, deputy director of the center, noted, there was a misunderstanding when the Americans first arrived in Iraq. Their assumption was that their mission was purely military, but now they understood that "cultural understanding is critical to prevail in the long war and to meet 21st century challenges. . . . We had the military tactics but lacked the knowledge of Iraqi laws and traditions so we needed to learn about them all" ("Coaching US Troops," 2007). At last, after four years, the importance of cultural training had struck home and was being addressed.

But the damage had already been done. By the time the center was set up, ignorance of etiquette regarding, for example, the force's treatment of local women, their use of search dogs, local hierarchies, and religious laws had already seen them break cultural norms with impunity and had helped destroy the chances of the United States being seen as an ally and not as an occupying force (Bordin, 2011). As of now, the United States, and in particular the troops, are still paying the price.

Such cultural ignorance or indifference often exacerbates our management of conflicts and wars (Park and Huang, 2010). Our ignorance is often not only about obviously important factors such as language and morality but also about how cultures conduct their relationships within their own group and with their authorities, their preferences for leadership styles, their styles of communication, and their attitudes toward gender and about themselves as part of a group. One of the greatest barriers to empathy and to being able to see another's group viewpoint is people's tendency to operate from a group-centric point of view (i.e., using one's own culture as the yardstick with which understand the world) and believing that one's own individual, social, and cultural characteristics are the right ones. While globalization is beginning to lessen such differences, it is extremely important that the differences that remain are taken into account, as differing cultures require varying and sensitive approaches to issues of engagement on, in particular, matters that are relevant to peacebuilding, where an own group-centric perspective can become a huge barrier to the work required (Vignoles et al., 2011).

Cultural Psychology and Cultural Neuroscience

Cultural psychology is the study of how cultures reflect and shape the psychological processes of their members (Ames and Fiske, 2010). More recently, the integration of theory and methods from social and cultural psychology and related bio-disciplines has given birth to a new field called "cultural neuroscience," which investigates how human brain functions are shaped by interactions between culture, brain, and genes (Han et al., 2013).

In recent years, brain imaging studies have uncovered variations in the neural substrates (i.e., the part of the central nervous system that underlies a specific behavior in differing cultures). Using brain imaging techniques has allowed researchers to access processes that are not readily available at the conscious level through self-reports (Lin and Telzer, 2018). It appears that our brains are biologically prepared to adapt to differing group contexts.

Scholars have noted evidence for differing cognitive processing styles such as perception, memory, perspective-taking, and attribution bias and for self-construal and empathy that can differ according to the sociocultural contexts in which individuals are brought up. Cultural traits can shape the occurrence of genomic, neurobiological, and psychological processes over time, and such processes, in turn, can facilitate even more complex social experiences and even broader behavioral processes (Chiao et al., 2010).

Why Such Differences?

Why are there such variations in the psychologic and genetic make-up of populations around the world? Gene–culture coevolution studies—also known as biocultural evolution or dual inheritance theory (Heinrich and McElreath, 2012)—suggest that while culture and genetics have traditionally been thought of as separate processes, researchers are now realizing that they may be closely connected, each influencing the natural progression of the other as genes and culture continually interact in a feedback loop (Goldman, 2014). According to culture–gene coevolutionary theory, differing cultural traits can possess an evolutionary advantage for a person or group. For instance, traits such as individualism and collectivism (Fincher et al., 2008) may serve adaptive functions, and thus culturally consistent differences may become selected for over successive generations, leading to population variation in the frequencies for certain genes.

Studies that compared the genomes of 150 Europeans from between 5,500 and 3,000 years ago with those of 305 modern Europeans descended from them have identified gene–culture coevolution in terms of health (e.g., milk tolerance, type 2 diabetes). It should therefore not surprise us that there should also be gene-culture co-evolution in terms of our mental an emotional processes (Rendell et al., 2011; see also Richerson and Boyd, 2005). These findings are supported by analyses of human genetic variation, which reveal that hundreds of genes have been subject to recent positive selection, often in response to human activities (Laland, Odling-Smee, and Myles, 2010). "Gene–culture dynamics are typically faster, stronger, and operate over a broader range of conditions than conventional evolutionary dynamics, leading some practitioners to argue that gene–culture co-evolution could be the dominant mode of human evolution" (Laland, Odling-Smee, and Myles, 2010, p. 137). It now appears that the human genome may be changing at an accelerating pace in response to population growth and new environments (Christakis, 2008; Creanza, Kolodny, and Feldman, 2017).

Geographical variability can actually predict cultural variability in such traits as individualism/collectivism. This may be because nations with a greater historical and contemporary rate of infectious diseases, such as malaria, typhus, or leprosy, are more likely to have adopted collectivistic cultural norms, possibly due to the anti-pathogen defense function that such norms may serve, by protecting vulnerable geographical regions from diseases (Chiao and Blizinsky, 2010; Fincher et al., 2008).

Genetic drift may also result in changes. Chen et al. (1999) discovered that relative to non-migratory populations, individuals from migratory populations possess a disproportionately higher frequency of a trait that influences dopamine signaling in brain circuits supporting novelty and sensation-seeking. Such traits may be a requirement in migratory societies as they can help people to succeed in the challenges of migration. Sedentary populations, on the other hand, may succeed not by exploring new environments but by developing intensive methods for using the limited amounts of land available (Netting, 1993). Within such sedentary societies, traits such as novelty-seeking and exploratory behaviors would be selected against.

As cultural traits become ever more complex in response to a rapidly changing world, it is likely that our usual cumulative cultural learning and its effects on traits will require ever more rapid learning between one generation and the next (Truskanov and Prat, 2018). Given the rapid rate of change today, it is difficult to establish just how much new trait learning is humanly possible. For the foreseeable future therefore it seems that peacebuilders will need to work on understanding the varied trait processes that differing communities have inherited and many still have. This is particularly important given that many such traits may actually be cultural mismatches with today's environments and are making the work on peacebuilding all the harder.

Cultural Dimensions of Behavior and Relationships

While there are many defined cultural differences between groups and nations (Hofstede, 2001), it is important to note (again!) that in today's globalizing world, many of these individual and societal characteristics are changing on account of greater interaction between cultures due to travel and the ever-increasing networks of entertainment, information, attitudes, and skills though widely available online processes.

High Culture versus Low Culture

Anthropologist Edward T. Hall first discussed high-context culture in his 1976 book *Beyond Culture*. He defined "high-context" cultures as societies or groups where people have been closely connected with each other over a long period of time, whereas "low context" refers to societies where people tend to have many connections but of shorter duration and where relationships are often built up for a specific reason.

In high-context societies, members often appear to implicitly know what the rules of interaction and behavior are, and these are rarely spelled out, which can make it difficult for outsiders to function optimally. High-context cultures usually include non-verbal methods in conversations—such as facial expressions, eye movements, and voice tones—which are often more important than the information conveyed by the words.

Authority is often more hierarchical in high-context cultures, and the bonds among people are often long-held and very strong. The development of trust between individuals and groups is also extremely important and can usually only develop over time—time, unfortunately, is not allocated often enough by low-context culture individuals and groups. Thus an individual from a low-context group can remain an outsider for a long time with a high-context group, and this can be a huge barrier to trust-building and productive peacebuilding. It is important to note that in high-context cultures people generally prefer to meet face to face rather than via technology and often prefer personal trust bonds over formal legal agreements.

In low-context cultures, information and relationships depend much more on language and explicit rules of behavior. Hierarchies are much flatter: in today's world, first names are becoming the norm, even to bosses. In a low-context culture, information is vested in the actual words people use and spelled out in an explicit manner and by being precise with spoken or written words, whereas very little is actually explicitly spelled out in high-context culture communications.

Such differences in trust in people, versus trust in written agreements, can be extremely frustrating for a mediator and other peacebuilders, as one party may want to invest time in the articulation of agreements, while the other party can see such requirements as a sign that they are not trusted.

Power Distance

Related to the concept of high-/low-context cultures is the issue of power distance. This term refers to the extent to which less powerful members of institutions and organizations within a culture expect and accept that power is distributed unequally (Hofstede, Hosfstede, and Minkov, 2010). A high power-distance culture accepts and maintains inequalities and a hierarchy of power and status more easily. In such a society, elders usually take the lead and are often regarded as role models and wise resources. Those seen as subordinate will usually defer to a higher-level person, and this deference will be accepted as natural by those on the higher level. On the contrary, in a low power-distance society, equality is often seen as the aim of society, and upward mobility is encouraged and common. In low power-distance cultures, every person expects to be listened to regardless of rank or background. These differences were investigated by Freeman et al. (2009), who scanned the brains of American and Japanese individuals to examine the differences in the neural display in relation to dominance and subordination. They found that activity in the right caudate nucleus of the brain, which plays an important role in how the brain learns and remembers, was correlated with behavioral tendencies of dominance versus subordination. The Americans self-reported a tendency toward more dominant behavior, whereas the Japanese self-reported a tendency toward more subordinate behavior—tendencies that were consistent with associated functional magnetic resonance imaging (fMRI) results. A misunderstanding on the part of the peacebuilder—for example, in knowing how to address people, or a lack of acknowledgment of hierarchies, and of who can speak first, and who actually holds the power in a room or on the field—can lead to many frustrated hours and a lack of agreement momentum on the part of the parties involved in the conflict. In addition, acceptance of inequalities within a society, as opposed to a more inclusive approach to issues of equity, can be a significant stumbling block to peacebuilding.

Individualism versus Collectivism

High- and low-context and power-distance characteristics are also intrinsically related to individualism and to its opposite, collectivism (i.e., the degree to which individuals see themselves as part of a group). This cultural dimension of individualism–collectivism has been shown to reliably affect a wide variety of human mental processes at a behavioral level, including self-concept, motivation, perception, emotion, and cognition (Markus and Kitayama, 1991; Triandis et al., 1988). This dimension has important influences on human emotions, ideas, and behaviors (Cross, Hardin, and Gercek-Swing, 2011) and the underlying brain mechanisms (Han and Northoff, 2008).

In a collectivistic culture, the focus is on the belief that the group is more important than an individual, which is shown through the use of conformity and consensus where possible. In collectivist cultures, individuals see themselves as highly interconnected and very much defined by their relations and by their social context. Individuals from interdependent cultures, such as Japan, tend to prize social harmony, conformity, and adherence to group norms (Ambady, 2011). Where collectivistic cultures dominate, people often care (or appear to care) more for group interests than an individual's. People consider people they are close to as integral parts of their self; they take responsibility for ingroup members and prefer group harmony and group development to competition (Nisbett et al., 2001). In contrast, people in individualistic cultures are rewarded for initiative, personal achievement, and showing leadership. When it comes to a conflict, they may feel freer to choose their individual preference on issues of conflict rather than that of their group.

> The United States, Canada, Australia, New Zealand, Israel, South Africa and most of the countries of Northern and Western Europe—except Portugal—are generally regarded as individualist societies.
>
> Argentina, Brazil, Chile, Colombia, Costa Rica, Ecuador, Egypt, El Salvador, Ethiopia, Ghana, Greece, Guatemala, Hong Kong, Indonesia, India, Iran, Iraq, Jamaica, Japan, Kenya, Kuwait, Lebanon, Libya, Malaysia, Mexico, Nigeria, Pakistan, Panama, Peru, Philippines, Portugal, Saudi Arabia, Sierra Leone, Singapore, South Korea, Taiwan, Tanzania, Thailand, Turkey, United Arab Emirates, Uruguay, Venezuela, former Yugoslavia, and Zambia are generally regarded as collectivist societies.

An awareness of how the differences and priorities of individualist or collectivist groups affect a party's or a nation's beliefs, practices, and ideologies is critical when attempting to develop accommodations between groups whose approaches differ.

Self-Construal

Self-construal refers to the extent to which the self is defined independently of others or interdependently with others. A wide range of studies, both Western- and Eastern-based, show Western independent views of the self as distinct from others, and Eastern interdependent views of the self as fundamentally related to others (Giacomin and Jordan, 2017). Westerners tend to view the self as a stable independent entity, whereas Easterners tend to construe the self in a more context-sensitive and relational manner. While Easterners view close others (and their relationships to those close others) as part of the self, Westerners tend to conceive of the self as an independent entity (Ames and Fiske, 2010). It appears that specific brain regions, such as the medial prefrontal cortex and posterior cingulate cortex are involved in this self-evaluation and self-knowledge (Amodio and Frith, 2006). Using cultural priming (i.e., presenting people with certain stimuli to make them think/feel/act like people of a certain culture) deepens such findings (Ng et al., 2010). Whereas Western cultures more often emphasize self-esteem and confidence in one's worth and abilities, in collectivistic cultures people more often strive to not lose face and to appear positively among social groups, and this has important consequences in all forms of dialogue, mediation, and strategy development for peacebuilding.

Again, it is important to note that such modes can shift depending on the environment and the pressures. Using fMRI, Chiao et al. (2010) found that, after being primed to think in an individualistic, "Western" manner, bicultural individuals showed greater self-referential brain activation for contextual versus general self-judgments, while bicultural individuals primed to think in a more collectivistic "Eastern" manner showed greater self-referential activation for contextual versus general self-judgments.

Uncertainty Avoidance

Uncertainty avoidance, as noted in Chapter 4 of this volume, deals with a person's tolerance for uncertainty and ambiguity and comfort or discomfort in unstructured or novel situations. A country with many people who have a high uncertainty avoidance will have a low tolerance for uncertainty and ambiguity. As a result, such a society is usually a conservative one and often very rule-oriented in terms of social norms, including religion. A low uncertainty-avoidance society is less concerned about ambiguity and uncertainty and has more tolerance of social variety and experimentation. It more readily accepts change and is more willing to take risks (Hofstede, 2001). In general, uncertainty avoidance scores are higher in East and Central European countries, in Latin countries, in Japan, and in German-speaking countries, while they are lower in English-speaking, Nordic, and Chinese-culture countries (Hofstede, 2011). Research suggests that people in uncertainty-avoiding countries are more likely to aspire to a unified appearance of truth, while uncertainty-accepting cultures are more tolerant of opinions different from those they are used to and are more relative in their opinions about the truth (Hofstede, 2011). Such biases need to be taken into account when structuring peacebuilding mediation, as constructive ambiguities, which are often an important part of peace agreements, can be more acceptable to one party than to the other.

Attribution Error

Cultures also differ in terms of attribution errors—that is, the tendency to explain people's behavior in terms of inherent personality traits rather than external, situational considerations (see Chapter 4 of this volume). It appears that Westerners are more inclined to focus attribution on personality factors, while Asians, for example, tend to reason more holistically by considering people's behavior in terms of their situation (Dean and Koenig, 2019; Mason and Morris, 2010). Thus, in a study of a crime, Western news focused on the person's innate character flaws and individual failings, while Chinese news pointed out the lack of relationships of the perpetrator in a foreign environment and the failings of society. South and East Asians also give more weight to the situational forces in explaining the causes of people's actions (Nisbett, 2003). Kobayashi, Glover, and Temple (2006) showed that Japanese participants exhibited greater activation in orbito-frontal regions of the cortex linked to thinking about others' beliefs than did American participants; that is, Japanese culture emphasizes greater attention to others' feelings relative to one's own.

Emotional Expression

Emotion regulation is the "processes by which individuals influence which emotions they have, when they have them, and how they experience and express these emotions' (Gross, 1998, p. 275). Culture shapes how people prefer to experience, express, recognize, and regulate their emotions (Mesquita and Leu, 2007). For example, it is common for leaders from the Middle East to accompany their expositions and regrets with tears, whereas such a display would be seen as a weakness in many Western countries (Butler, Lee, and Gross, 2007). Using cross-cultural fMRI neuroimaging, Chiao (2009) discovered a cultural variation effect in bilateral amygdala responses to emotional scenes between Japanese American and Caucasian American participants.

It appears that behavioral perception of emotional expressions may affect the neural response to emotional expressions as well. For example, Derntl et al. (2009) reported that Asian immigrants to Austria showed a significant response to the emotional facial expressions of Caucasians (i.e., expressions of anger and disgust) but that the strength of this response was negatively correlated with the amount of time they had been in the foreign culture, showing, once again, how differences can be ameliorated with familiarity and over time.

Gender Constraints

Gender still plays a huge role, as seen in the non-acceptance of women as useful peacebuilders, particularly at the elite level (Council on Foreign Relations, n.d.). This is not surprising given that women's voices are still missing from the most branches of governments and parliaments worldwide. Only 24.3 percent of all national parliamentarians were women as of February 2019, a slow increase from 11.3 percent in 1995 (UN Women, 2019). This lack of women's equal participation in societal matters has significant consequences for peacebuilding. It appears that countries that display lower levels of gender equality are more likely to become involved in civil conflict, and the violence is likely to be greater, than in countries where women have a higher status (Forsberg and Olsson, 2016). Unfortunately, women are also still much less likely to be seated at a peace agreement table— despite the evidence suggesting that when women are included in negotiations, the agreement is 35 percent more likely to endure for at least fifteen years (Inclusive Security, n.d.).

It can be a challenge for those of us working in the field who have to, as I did, at times refuse a leadership role in a peacebuilding process in a country where women were generally disregarded because of my assessment that a man's presence would be more effective and would make the process more successful. This is beginning to change but slowly. In the meantime, it is important to be aware of how understanding gender culture is critical to successfully strategizing peacebuilding in conflict situations and hopefully, as an add-on, increasing the visibility and active peacebuilding roles of women.

According to Hofstede and Fink (2007), masculinity score denotes the degree to which societies reinforce, or do not reinforce, the traditional masculine role models of achievement, control, and power; a low masculinity score means a society has a lower level of differentiation and a high level of inequity between genders (ChangeFactory, n.d.). Countries differ in their bias toward such masculinity. Such biases can easily be ascertained by checking out countries in the Hofstede Country Comparison chart (Hofstede Insights, n.d.). In one of his studies, Hofstede presented masculinity versus femininity index scores for 76 countries, noting that masculinity is high in Japan, in German-speaking countries, and in some Latin countries like Italy and Mexico; it is moderately high in English-speaking Western countries; it is low in Nordic countries and in the Netherlands; and moderately low in Latin and Asian countries such as France, Spain, Portugal, Chile, Korea, and Thailand (Hofstede, 2011). More recently, Kachel, Steffens, and Niedlich (2016) developed a self-perceived masculinity/femininity scale, which permits a greater variety of gender self-ascription; however, many such ascriptions are consistent with the Hofstede scale.

Taking account of such beliefs and social perceptions about the varying roles that men/women can play (while stretching them if possible) can be important in successful peacebuilding. It can also be useful to utilize existing stereotypes of women (while waiting for them to change!), such as their being less threatening to men in many situations and therefore often able to carry out discussions/shuttle mediations etc. where such are needed but are too problematic for the men to undertake (Fitzduff, 2010, 2013).

The Role of Religion

For many communities, their cultural identities and their religious belief systems and practices are inextricably linked, thus making clear boundaries between cultural and spiritual/religious heritage, tradition, and expression difficult to delineate (Holt and Machnyikova, 2013, p. 179). These religious values are what are called "sacred values"—that is, "any value that a moral community implicitly or explicitly treats as possessing infinite or transcendental significance that precludes comparisons, trade-offs, or indeed any other mingling with bounded or secular values" (Tetlock et al., 2000, p. 853). The intricacies of conflicts with such a religious value dimension can be even more difficult to resolve than normal identity conflicts, since it is hard for groups to reconcile unquestionable beliefs and behaviors with those of others, given that such beliefs and behaviors are often part of their whole way of life and the actual ascribed meaning of their lives. Christian concepts such as some people being religiously "saved" (i.e., having received reassurance from a God of a relationship with God and a promise of eternal life in heaven with God) and others who are not "saved" can significantly influence a group's capacity for joint respect and positive dialogue and peacebuilding. Similarly, a perception of all who are not Muslims as being "kafir" or infidels can undermine societal and intergroup peacebuilding. A religious framework that validates caste—such as the Dalits in relation to Hindus in India—can seriously affect discussions of issues of respect and resources. Buddhists' concepts of sacred nationalism in Sri Lanka can limit their capacity for inclusive peacebuilding with their Hindu and Muslim neighbors. The concept of Jerusalem as sacred to both Jews and Muslims has been a downfall for any agreements between them during many decades of conflict.

Many of the issues addressed in this chapter are important to all work that involves a religious dimension. Hierarchies, the role of individual thinking, and people's capacity to deal with uncertainties, gender stereotypes, and self-construal—all of these must be examined in addition to the belief systems that need to be taken into account. There have been many years of interfaith work that have produced interesting models, which have been tailored to suit particular contexts where such "sacred values" are a factor (USAID, 2009).

An important extra perspective to bring to inter-religious peacebuilding work is the research outlined in Chapter 4 of this book, which notes that belief systems (including religion) are not usually about the veracity of "truths" but much more a buy-in into particular communities of belonging, with all the positives and negatives that that can bring. Thus religious beliefs (and many other ideologies) are about meaning, about being part of a group, about certainty and security, and about status and respect, all of which are also important to recognize before interfaith work can be successful. It is useful to have buy-in from religious leaders who are trusted fellow "believers" but are able to, for example, stretch sacred books' interpretations to allow for the inclusion of other groups as equally human. Providing safe opportunities and a comfortable emotional state for believers' encounters with those of other beliefs is also particularly important for interfaith work.

Conclusion

The previously discussed ideas are based on the assumption that there can be a continuum of all these processes within a society and between groups. It is also assumed that individuals can acquire more than one set of cultural knowledge and can use different sets depending on the cues from the contexts in which they live and work (Han et al., 2013). Exposing individuals to particular cultural symbols may also activate specific cultural knowledge and result in mindsets and behaviors that are consistent with that culture. For instance, it appears that bicultural individuals can often switch between Western and East Asian cultural mindsets.

There is also evidence that neurological activations can be changed as a function of adapting to or learning from a new culture (Hedden et al., 2008). It seems that even a temporary, incidental exposure to another culture can change the brain activation pattern when performing the same cognitive task at different times and in different contexts. This implies that whereas individuals inherit or develop a habitual pattern of neurological behaviors, following chronic (repeated) exposure to a certain culture, the brain retains its capacity to adapt to new cultural influence (Park and Huang, 2010). Thus it appears that learning can change not only our thoughts and behaviors but also (somewhat!) our physiologies. It is therefore important that, while remaining cognizant of cultural variability in thought and affective processes throughout the world, one does not assume outdated stereotypes regarding differences in behaviors, communication styles, trust norms, gender, etc., given a rapidly integrating world in which emigration and social media are continually flattening out traditional differences.

8

New Horizons, New Tribes

No technology has been weaponized at such an unprecedented global scale as social media.

—Ong and Cabañes (2018)

We are in a battle, and more than half of this battle is taking place in the battlefield of the media.

—Ayman al-Zawahiri, then al-Qaeda's second-in-command (2005)

The crowd becomes one vast neural network through which sentiments travel from body to body at ultra high speed.

—W. Davies (2018, p. 11)

Introduction

In mid-2016 the Sudanese president and his vice-president had settled into an uneasy truce after years of civil war when a false Facebook message said the vice-president had been arrested: the ensuing battle left three hundred dead and plunged the nation back into conflict (Mach, 2016).

The Islamic State of Iraq and the Levant (ISIL) sources funds by using Instagram, Facebook, and YouTube and asks for donations via PayPal (Singer and Brooking, 2018, p. 65). ISIL leaders have even promoted their dissemination of propaganda as a form of worship (Winter, 2017). In Libya, Facebook is used by "keyboard warriors" as an arena through which conflicting Libyans utilize violent rhetoric, coordinate their attacks on each other, and spread fake news (D. Walsh and Zway, 2018). In Myanmar, Buddhist nationalists have used social media, particularly Facebook, to stoke fear about Muslims and the ethnic Rohingya, who are promoted as enemies of Buddhism or of the State (Miles, 2018). Hezbollah ran and equipped a mujahid campaign on Facebook and Twitter that allowed supporters to fulfill their religious

Our Brains at War. Mari Fitzduff, Oxford University Press (2021). © Oxford University Press.
DOI: 10.1093/oso/9780197512654.003.0009

obligations by buying weapons and ammunition for the war (Singer and Broking, 2018, p. 65). In Sri Lanka, rumors depicting Muslims as plotting to sterilize and ultimately wipe out the Sinhalese have increased deadly protests and revenge attacks throughout the country (Guyon, 2018). In Nigeria, Boko Haram uses YouTube videos to encourage its members to kill those who refuse Allah: "Brethren, wherever you are, I pray this meets you well. I give you the go ahead, whether you are two or three, take up your weapons and start killing them . . . all those who refuse Allah. . . . Kill kill and kill (Malefakis, 2019). In 2016 an Iraqi militia captured a suspected ISIL fighter and then invited 75,000 online fans to vote on whether to kill or release him. The fans voted to kill him, and the militia posted the video with a caption saying thanks for the vote. In other words, "a guy on the toilet in Omaha, Nebraska, could emerge from the bathroom with the blood of some 18-year-old Syrian on his hands" (Singer and Brooking, 2018, p. 66). In January 2021, after the storming of the United States Capitol in Washington D.C. by supporters of President Trump, both Facebook and Twitter paused the account of the president saying that his use of it was incentivating violence.

The Weaponization of Social Media

Much has been written about the changing nature of the hardware of war, as new technologies such as drones, lasers, unmanned fighting vehicle, long-range artillery, and hypersonic missiles transform the ways in which future wars will be fought. Less has been written about the ways in which our human software, which has been optimized for a very different environment than that of today, will respond to the impact of the Internet and, in particular, to the interactive social media platforms that are already transforming war and peacebuilding issues.

Platforms such as Facebook, Twitter, and YouTube have changed how people, communities, and nations relate to each other, form new connections, or deepen older ones. Unfortunately, many of the changes are negative for peacebuilding in that they have been used to deepen hostilities rather than understanding within and between groups, societies, and nations. As Mercy Corps (2019) has noted, social media has

created new, highly accessible channels for spreading disinformation, sowing divisiveness and contributing to real-world harm in the form of violence, persecution and exploitation. The impact social media has on real-world communities is complex and rapidly evolving. It stretches across international borders and challenges traditional humanitarian aid, development and peacebuilding models.

What Are Social Media Platforms?

Social media comprises interactive computer-mediated technological platforms that facilitate the creation and sharing of information and ideas via virtual online communities and networks. These include Facebook, YouTube, Twitter, Instagram, WeChat, QQ, QZone, Weibo, Twitter, Tumblr, Reddit, etc. The major platforms currently being used in weaponizing war are Facebook, Twitter, and YouTube. Their reach is unparalleled in human history. As of December 2019, roughly 510,000 comments were posted on Facebook every minute, and in 2019 Facebook was estimated to have over 2.5 billion users (Hutchinson, 2020) using 111 languages (Fick and Dave, 2019). YouTube has over 2 billion users, with 5 billion videos watched per day, and over 400 hours of video uploaded to it every minute. It covers 95 percent of the Internet population (Chi, 2019). Twitter hosts 500 million tweets every day and is the number one platform for government leaders (Cooper, 2019). It has a total of 1.3 billion accounts, with 320 million monthly active users, and its platform functions in eighty languages (Aslam, 2020; K. Smith, 2020).

"Bad Actors"

Facebook had a very hopeful start. It was originally designed specifically to connect people, and its success in doing this has been unprecedented. It was hoped that through such communication it could also enhance democracy by making it easier for people to discuss issues, organize around causes, and participate actively in democratic processes. Its design made it possible for such ideas to be shared in an interactive way, which was impossible for more passive traditional media such as TV and radio. Supporters of such hopes believed that social media could create what economists call "a positive supply-side shock" to the amount of freedom in the world (Shirky, 2019).

This prognosis was partially right, and the democratization processes of the Arab Spring that began in 2011 would not have happened without social media (Mitchell, Brown, and Guskin, 2012). But in the past few years, many began to ask questions about whether or not social media was helping or hindering social and global understanding (Carr, 2015). The 2016 elections in the United States and the Brexit campaign abounded in "fake news" and proliferated processes whose purpose seemed to be to subvert democracy. Despite initial denials, Facebook itself finally admitted that it was being used in unforeseen ways with societal and political repercussions that were never anticipated. "In 2016, we at Facebook were far too slow to recognize how bad actors were abusing our platform" (Harbath, 2018).

Many such "bad actors" were pursuing their own particular conflict and war interests, often in opposition to peacebuilding efforts. The work of many conflict agencies and development agencies is being skewed by a variety of social media processes that are detrimental ways to the purposes of peacebuilding. According to Mercy Corps (2019), these include

- *Information operations.* Coordinated disinformation campaigns designed to disrupt and confuse decision making, create social divisions, and delegitimize adversaries.
- *Political manipulation.* Campaigns that are used to systematically manipulate political discussions within a state and between states. This includes distorting news reporting, silencing dissenters, and undermining democratic governance and electoral systems.
- *Digital hate speech.* Social media platforms amplify and disseminate hate speech, thus helping individuals and groups to use and prey on existing fears and grievances.
- *Radicalization and recruitment.* Social media processes are used by violent extremists and militant organizations to recruit new members.

Warfare on the Internet has become an integral part of modern conflict operations. War can now be fought in a virtual form in which anyone with an Internet connection can affect the outcome of any election and any conflict. Those who control the platforms of the Internet are skewing and often winning both political power and the world's wars.

Given the social significance of such platforms, and their apparent capacity to influence the emotions, beliefs, and behavior of individuals and groups, neuroscientists are now studying social media's effects on the brain and how neural systems support and interact with social media usage (Curley and Ochsner, 2017; Meshi, Tamir, and Heekeren, 2015). While such platforms arise and develop at an increasingly rapid rate, it appears that we ourselves remain all too human, with many of our evolved and inherited emotions and social responses still basically affecting the ways in which we interact with social media platforms and are influenced by them.

Deliberate Enticement

It now appears that at least part of the capacity for "bad actors" to utilize social media for their own particular interests, whether economic or political, arises because of the very ways in which social media sustains itself financially. The profit for social media companies comes from their harvesting of personal information by collecting data on people about what they like, want, and believe, based on their online activity, interests, gender, sexual preference, geographical location, religion, and social media posts. Such information allows advertisers to tailor their ads through psychometric profiling of potential customers. The more data these platforms can collect, the more profitable it is for the social media companies, and they are therefore deliberately designed to be addictive. Analysts can create psychologically addictive programs based on personal profiles that they harness through their surveillance of usage, and they can then sell this information to political actors and others with interests in persuading and manipulating the public toward specific goals (Vaidhyanathan, 2018). One example is Cambridge Analytica, a British political consulting firm that combined "misappropriation of digital assets, data mining, data brokerage and data analysis with strategic communication during the electoral processes" (Ingram, 2018).

Why Are Social Media Platforms
So Influential?

Preliminary research appears to show that platforms like Facebook, Snapchat, and Instagram excite the very same neural circuitry that is also used by slot machines and by cocaine to keep enticing people to come back again and again to their products as much as possible. Magnetic resonance imaging (MRI) scans illustrate that feedback via social media activates the reward center of the brain in a way that is similar to addictive drugs (Sherman et al., 2016). The human brain contains four major dopamine pathways that act as highways for chemical messengers called neurotransmitters and as connections between different parts of the brain. Three of these pathways—the mesocortical, mesolimbic, and nigrostriatal pathways—are considered our "reward pathways," which are responsible for the release of dopamine in various parts of the brain and are involved in most cases of addiction. Although not as intense as, for example, a hit of drugs, positive social stimuli will similarly result in a release of dopamine. Because of its endless nature, social media will provide us with a virtually unlimited supply of such stimuli. "Every notification, whether it's a text message, a 'like' on Instagram, or a Facebook notification, has the potential to be a positive social stimulus and dopamine influx" (Haynes, 2018).

In this regard, MRI scans have indicated that social networking site addiction is similar in terms of brain anatomy alterations to other substance addictions (He, Turel, and Bechara, 2017). Cognitive neuroscientists have shown that rewarding social stimuli recognition such as laughing faces by our peers and messages from loved ones activate the same dopaminergic reward pathways as alcohol or drugs (Haynes, 2018). By its nature, which limits messages to 280 (formerly 140) characters, Twitter is even more addictive, as the dopamine system is most powerfully stimulated when the information coming in is so small that it doesn't fully satisfy. "A short text or tweet . . . is ideally suited to send your dopamine system raging" (Weinschenk, 2012).

Social networking sites grab our attention because they are often designed to involve self-relevant information, and they also have a bearing on our social status and reputation. This reward circuitry is thought to be particularly sensitive in adolescence, and it could help explain why teenagers are avid social media users. The power of social platforms has been exponentially increased by the use of bots—automated applications designed to amplify messages and programmed to mimic natural human interactions such as liking, commenting, following, and unfollowing on social media platforms. Chatbots—bots designed to stimulate conversations with human users in ways that make it difficult for users to differentiate between human and automated interactions—have become ubiquitous and influential in democracy processes and in political and social conflicts.

Social Media, War, and Neuroscience

It now appears that many of the social and neural processes identified in the previous chapters in this book are likely to be magnified by social media as these new forms of communication create new kinds of conflict and become a magnet for existing ones. By and large, social media processes often multiply emotions at the expense of reason, provide specious opportunities for meaning and belonging, and facilitate the dissemination of fake news at the expense of evidence-based beliefs (Tactical Tech, 2018).

The Multiplication of Emotion

Critical thinking to determine fact from fiction and to ensure appropriate problem-solving generally takes place in the frontal cortex of the brain. Managing the multiplicity of individual and group societal needs and creating solutions to improve the social good of all citizens is critical to the creation of sustainable and peaceful societies. In such management, balancing reason and emotion is essential. An ability to rise above the emotions of particular groups and govern in an inclusive and fair fashion is essential if peace is to be sustained. Unfortunately, in the midst of the chaos and disturbance that attends most conflicts, more primitive and emotion-based neurological systems tend to take over. As noted in previous chapters, the two regions of the brain that struggle for attention are the amygdala (the part of the brain that processes our automatic/intuitive emotional impulses) and the prefrontal cortex (which deals with our conscious/reasoned/logical responses to a situation). These "emotional" and "reasoning" minds coexist particularly uneasily in situations of conflict.

Electroencephalography and hormonal testing reveal that in any perceived conflict situation we are at the mercy of our amygdala's response, given its critical role in detecting fear and preparing our bodies for an emergency reaction to a possibly threatening situation. Stress hormones like adrenaline and cortisol flood our system, preparing us for fight or for flight. Unfortunately, it turns out that social media platforms exaggerate these tendencies as they often speak directly to the "most reactive, least reflective parts of our minds, demanding we pay attention even when our calmer selves might tell us not to" (Golumbia, 2018). Thus fearful and angry posts seem to stimulate biochemical responses that make people anxious and more likely to share these posts with others and thus ensure that anger is the emotion that travels fastest into the social networks (Fan, Xu, and Zhao, 2016). In addition, individuals with larger online social networks have larger amygdalae than individuals with smaller social networks (X. Liu et al., 2018).

Given the designed ability of social media platforms to attract attention for commercial, social, or political causes, their algorithms prioritize posts that contain strong emotions and will facilitate their spreading of them to others. Research by the *Wall Street Journal* discovered that YouTube's algorithms more often recommended "conspiracy theories, partisan viewpoints and misleading videos" over more reputable but "boring" videos representing fact-based reporting (Nicas, 2018). Unfortunately, often the more partisan a person is, the more followers they will attract on social media (Edkins, 2017). Our human social and neurological tendencies and needs can therefore easily be hijacked by those who seek to use social media to deleteriously affect others, and we become easy prey for leaders and other purveyors of conflict who wish to persuade us to support particular goals or objectives. Such prioritizing of feelings makes it harder for reason to get a hold in deciding negative or positive judgments about group, religious, ethnic, racial, and national characteristics and possible relationships. Thus given that emotions, particularly fearful emotions, are often strong and contagious online, it can be easily seen how a dedicated group of social media savvies can incite a war. If a radio was sufficient to help launch a genocide in Rwanda, how much more easily could a genocide be launched with today's social media?

Twitter and Facebook have actually demonstrated the power of their platforms to manipulate their users' emotions by changing their news feed. In 2014 Facebook published details of a vast experiment in which it manipulated information posted on 689,000 users' home pages and found it could make people feel more positive or negative through a process of "emotional contagion" (Booth, 2014). As Davies (2018, p. 13) has noted, the contemporary notion of "viral marketing" is an example of systematically employed contagions. Such power to promote emotional contagion is unprecedented, and it has potentially disastrous consequences if used by the wrong hands in situations of tension and violence.

The Human Need for Significance

As noted in Chapters 3 to 5 of this book, the need to have some significance in our lives is universal. Social media interactive platforms provide new ways for people to find such meaning through giving them causes they can support and a way to participate in activities that will result in them being accepted and well liked. Using social media and achieving apparent acceptance of ourselves and our views can cause a widespread reaction across our brains' reward center.

At the University of California–Los Angeles Ahmanson-Lovelace Brain Mapping Center, researchers used functional MRI to see exactly how teenagers' brains were lit up when their photos received "likes." It was reported that "the brain fires off shots of dopamine as people posted, reposted, and expressed their likes or dislikes and ideas" (Wolpert, 2016). Thus, our brains become addicted to the images and feelings that are invoked by our social media interactions in a way that is similar to addictive drugs (i.e., as a means of feedback that shapes reinforcement learning). Providing "likes" to others on social media creates activation in brain circuitry that is implicated in reward, including the striatum and ventral tegmental area, regions that are also implicated in the experience of receiving "likes" from others (Sherman et al., 2018).

No Need to Be an Outsider

Social media interactions can also often offer an effective cure to loneliness. Nowadays, a person can often acquire shots of dopamine and oxytocin through participation in social media networks more easily than in real life. The evolved human brain often fails to recognize the difference between what is seen on the screen and real live people. Thus, for example, Facebook can easily fool our brain into thinking we are members of particular groups and thus increase the neural rewards for group connections.

A major problem, however, is that spending too much time on social media activates herd mentality; that is, people may lose their ability to think for themselves and form their own opinions because they are more likely to go along with what's most popular. As groups of like-minded people clump together, they grow to resemble "fanatical tribes, trapped in echo chambers of their own design" (Singer and Brooking, 2018, p. 123). These "social media bubbles" or "echo chambers" have huge implications for conflict, empowering attitudes and "facts" to deepen societal cleavages.

Our temporoparietal junction—an area of the brain that incorporates information from the thalamus and from the limbic system and orients our attention—is activated significantly more when dealing with apparently successful viral ideas. We automatically gravitate toward ideas or people that have a cachet of success. Functional MRI studies show increased activation in the visual cortex of the brain when viewing a photo with a significant number of likes versus the same photo with only a few likes (Sherman et al., 2018). This suggests that our brains intuitively pay more attention to something that has been arbitrarily rated better socially, regardless of the rational content.

Before social media, a group like ISIL had little opportunity to communicate or recruit members outside of its own territory. This capacity increased exponentially when it harnessed the power of social media. During its heyday, ISIL used social media to share three videos, fifteen photographic reports, and between 46,000 and 70,000 pro-ISIL Twitter posts every day to fuel the excitement and loyalty of its social media followers (Radsch, 2016). This helps explain the successful recruitment of groups such as ISIL who used social media to establish their cause as a heroic and inspirational one to which many young men—and some women—responded. A significant decline in the social media output of ISIL may help explain the decreasing number of volunteers now setting out from Western countries to join in the building of the caliphate. Without its success cachet—given the fact that the caliphate is now an apparently failing venture—its attraction is significantly diminished ("Analysis," 2017).

Youth in particular are significant users of social media. The need to belong to a group, to have meaning, and to be respected is particularly pertinent among adolescents, as noted in Chapter 5 of this volume. Given such biophysical rewards such as dopamine and oxytocin available freely from interaction with the Internet, it is no wonder that many are vulnerable to extremism. Social media has thus revolutionized the increase in militia memberships, particularly in the Middle East and parts of Africa, and has helped swell the revival of nationalism and the far right around the world. Groups such as white supremacist groups in the United States, Germany, and other countries rely heavily on social media to recruit and organize their members, using primarily sites like Facebook and Twitter as well as some that allow anonymity, like Reddit, YouTube, 4chan, and 8chan. The Southern Poverty Law Center (2019) has designated 1,020 US organizations as hate groups, all of whom are utilizing social media to purvey their work. This figure is the highest in at least twenty years.

Truth Is as We See It

As we have seen in Chapter 4 of this volume, truth is often more about our needs than about facts. In social media any resemblances to reality and to truth are often left far behind and replaced with tweaked, twisted, or imagined narratives. The human brain was never equipped to operate in an information environment that moves at the speed of the Internet. Our brains use shortcuts to filter almost all of the information that we receive—if they did not, we'd be completely overwhelmed and unable to pick out what information is useful at any particular moment (Colgin et al., 2009). Thus, often lacking the time or energy to investigate complex issues in depth, we use an "availability heuristic (i.e., a mental shortcut to help us arrive at a decision more quickly; Tversky and Kahneman, 1974). Our attention span is a finite commodity, and fascist leaders and dubious militias are increasingly adept at gaining attention through social media.

Given the overwhelming information available to us on the web and via social media, we can easily be confused and led astray in our decisions. Our brains are often just not capable of deciding what is true and worthy of reading and what is just noise or garbage. For many users, all information acquired on the web now has the same status, with no hierarchy of truth. Without an understanding of the differing quality of sources, reputable news or reports often have no more value than fabricated propaganda content on social media, and it is much harder for nuances of belief or affiliation to prevail in many of the networks purveying such information. The like/dislike of YouTube and the tweet and retweet of Twitter are usually about empathizing with your online buddies, not your responses to reading informed reports on an issue. The result is that there is often no longer a set of common "facts" upon which to base decisions; instead there exists a set of "opinions" or "fake news" for every conceivable point of view. To compound such availability, "fake news" penetrates, further, faster, and deeper into the social network than accurate information (Vosoughi, Roy, and Aral, 2018). Because of the algorithms attendant on such news feeds, social media platforms filter and display the news content likely to match users' group or political preferences.

Thus, receiving news from social media can increase all forms of polarization due to users having little interaction with those whose beliefs are different from their own. Recent research has demonstrated that social media has the power to increase the scope of stereotypes in people of all ages (Mihailidis and Viotty, 2017). A groups comes to believe that only its own members know the "truth" and that all others are ignorant, biased, and/or evil. Conspiracy theories flourish on the Internet and offer their believers a satisfying sense of having special access to a "truth." Thus divisions and hatreds become much easier, conspiracy theories flourish more freely, and conflicts and wars are more easily developed and more difficult to manage and end. At the end of 2015, the *Washington Post* quietly ended a weekly feature devoted to debunking ill-informed Internet conspiracy theories, admitting there were simply too many of them to note.

Enemies at a Click

Although originally designed to provide new and universal opportunities for people to "belong" to different social networks, many social media platforms now assist people and groups to practice the art of "othering" at local and global levels. The social media spreaders of conflict, hate, and war—as noted in the examples at the beginning of this chapter—are so far outsmarting the best efforts of governments, major societal institutions, and the peacebuilding profession. The Internet has become a battlefield that is freely available to authoritarian leaders and hate-mongering groups. As personal and group goals and emotions can now be shared globally, constituencies can be as wide as the world. Thus, social media effectively multiplies the capacity for individuals and groups to divide, compete, and conflict with each other, and its use appears to be increasing the number of warring militia factions around the world (Walter, 2017). Formerly, most militias depended on local or national support to make mobilization possible. The Internet has increased the possibilities for militia funding, as well as providing a way for militias to promote their cause and increase recruitment for their wars (Jacobson, 2010).

Social media harm is not confined to openly warring countries. During the 2016 US election campaign, social media processes constructed what are called filter bubbles around their users, fed them false claims, and smeared opponents by retweeting articles from low-credibility sources (Ciampaglia and Menczer, 2018). Twitter has admitted that more than 50,000 Russia-linked accounts used its service to post automated material about the 2016 US election. The company said the posts had reached at least 677,775 Americans (Swaine, 2018). Many of these were part of a botnet, a software application that runs automated tasks over the Internet at a much higher rate than would be possible for a human alone (P. Handley, 2018). Thousands of click farms (businesses that pay employees to click on website elements to artificially boost the status of a social or political idea) existed and still exist. Nowhere was this more evident than in the US election campaign of 2016, where a troll army helped steer the debates online by the use of chatbots masquerading as people. Accounts were unceasingly built and rebuilt to influence the stories and trends that could increase confusion and blur the line between assertions and facts. The UK Brexit campaign was similarly distorted by the use of social media (Hänska and Bauchowitz, 2017).

Conclusion

As the reach of social media increases, we are looking at a future of algorithmic manipulations with the power to determine the "success" or "failure" of a peacebuilding operation. Unfortunately, fighting an army of digital conspiracists is extremely difficult. Psychologists have discovered that trying to fight confirmation bias by demonstrating people's errors often makes the problem worse and deepens bias (Weir, 2017). The result is that war, tech, and politics have blurred into a new kind of battlespace that plays out on our smartphones and laptops for our emotions, and neither technological experts nor politicians, nor academics nor non-governmental organizations know for certain yet how to successfully challenge the trend, although some are trying to do so (see Chapter 10 of this volume).

Innovations in information and communications have long been feared. Socrates feared the written word as the beginning of a societal downfall; the first printing press was regarded similarly. The difference today is the scale and speed of the Internet. Unfortunately, because of the rate at which we humans can assimilate information and our often maladaptive neurological responses to social media, as noted in this chapter, as a species we as yet appear to be biologically and psychologically ill equipped to handle the instantaneity and the immensity of information that defines our social media age.

But, for better or for worse, we now live in a world where most citizens operate in an interactive Internet environment. Almost 4.54 billion people were active Internet users as of January 2020, encompassing 59 percent of the global population (Statista, 2020). These numbers are certain to increase over the coming decades. Like it or not, social media is now a major player—in some ongoing battles *the* major player—in all of our conflicts, both domestic and international. How to ensure that it can better serve our peacebuilding purposes by delivering on what is the best in our human biosocial nature, and not the worst, is a major question for the decades ahead.

9

The Next Adaptation?

Human beings are intrinsically social. Our survival critically depends on social interactions with others, the formation of alliances
and accurate social judgments.

—Decety and Lamm (2014)

Human prosociality is at the heart of peaceful societies and it is key
to facing global challenges.

—Böckler et al. (2018)

Introduction

In the Rwanda genocide of 1994, many Hutu Muslims protected Tutsi
Muslims and non-Muslims, sometimes losing their own lives in the process.
No Muslim religious leaders were charged or arrested for participating in the
genocide, and no one who sought refuge at mosques was killed with the col-
lusion of the Muslim leadership. This was in contrast to a trend across the
country whereby those seeking safety at Christian churches and state offices
were often killed at the order of, or with the cooperation of, religious and
state leaders. People who died at mosques were killed despite the active resistance of Muslims and non-Muslims protecting them.

The president of Rwanda made a public statement in 1995 in recognition of the Muslim community's positive behavior, at a ceremony cele-
brating the appointment of the first Muslim member of cabinet (minister).
He said that Muslims in Rwanda did not participate in the genocide and
called on them to "teach other Rwandans how to live together" (Doughty
and Ntambara, 2005).

Was the behavior of the Muslim community natural or unnatural?

Our Brains at War. Mari Fitzduff, Oxford University Press (2021). © Oxford University Press.
DOI: 10.1093/oso/9780197512654.003.0010

Beyond Ourselves?

Charles Darwin viewed altruism and cooperation with non-kin people or groups as a perplexing challenge to his theory of natural selection. Altruism and cooperative behavior, which can increase the fitness of a non-kin recipient at the expense of the giving individual, appear to contradict his belief that natural selection favors the evolution of behaviors that enhance the survival of the individual and their family. However, altruism is common, as a glance around the modern world will indicate (Klein, 2011). According to Fehr and Fischbacher (2004a), "human societies represent a spectacular outlier with respect to all other animal species because they are based on large-scale cooperation among genetically unrelated individuals" (p. 142). As humans, we appear to have attained an unparalleled level of complexity in certain forms of collaborative and cooperative activities (Apicella and Silk, 2019). It appears that the scope and the extent of such human cooperation has been and must be critical to the development of large-scale processes such as nation-building and international, global security, and economic institutions. So why has such cooperative behavior developed?

The Need to Cooperate

There is a very vigorous debate among researchers as to when and whether the individual gene for survival will override group needs. While the theory for the success of individual genes—the so-called selfish gene theory (Dawkins, 1976)—has been well addressed, the suggestion that there is a biological tendency toward cooperation, and the altruism needed for it, is relatively new. It was only in 2010 that the famous biologist E. O. Wilson and a team of colleagues at Harvard concluded that altruism had evolved for the good of the community rather than for the good of individual genes (Bergland, 2012). Noting the prevalence of cooperation and its importance, Wilson suggested that the human race had attained its superpowers by "being super-cooperators, groupies of the group, willing to set aside our small, selfish desires and I-minded drive to join forces and seize opportunity as a self-sacrificing, hive-minded tribe" (Angier, 2012). His research indicated that the individual and their close family are not in fact always the most important in terms of survival theories, but that altruism expands beyond them to protect other individuals in other social groups, whether or not they are related (Nowak, Tarnita, and Wilson, 2010).

It appears that in the process that was evolution, cooperation became increasingly important for group members' own survival. Thus people who were able to hunt and forage well together were much more likely to succeed and to defend themselves against threats from outside the tribe (Sullivan, 2016; Tomasello et al., 2012). As groups became more aware of the advantages of larger groups, they merged with other groups to expand their capacities, thus proving that human beings are capable of transcending their tribalistic instincts to further a common goal (Radovanović, 2019). In fact, the research seems to suggest that cooperative and altruistic behaviors are not just by-products of competition but they are actually the essential ingredients in evolution and development (Weiss and Buchanan, 2009). It appears that our long-term survival as humans has been predicated on our willingness to share information, resources, and help with others beyond our tribe. Our tendencies for altruism and cooperation appear to be an available glue that underlies the ability that humans have for living together in larger groups. These tendencies seem to be both hard-wired and social—that is, they are very dependent on the cultural norms of societies where altruism and prosocial behavior such as cooperation are normalized and institutionalized.

Sharing from Childhood

The skills and motivation to engage in complex forms of collaboration and cooperation seem to emerge early in infancy and childhood. Bloom (2013) documented sensitivity to fairness and reciprocity in babies as young as three months old. It appears that children will help each other from as early as 14 months of age, and from their second year of life, children can solve simple problems collaboratively (Tomasello and Hamann, 2012; Warneken and Tomasello, 2010). At three years, children show strong indications of conforming to the norm and being happy with the punishment of uncooperative individuals. The evolutionary trait that makes the survival of the infant dependent on the caring of not just their parents but also other relatives (Berlatsky, 2014) may have assisted such behavior, which appears to have emerged as a distinctly human combination of innate and learned behaviors.

However, the extent of cooperation varies across societies, as noted by House et al. (2013), who examined prosocial behaviors (i.e., behaviors intended to benefit others). The study of 326 children aged three to four-teen years and 120 adults from six societies spanned a wide range of cul-ture, geography, and subsistence strategies, including foragers, herders, horticulturalists, and urban dwellers across the Americas, Oceania, and Africa.

House et al. (2013) discovered that the rates of prosocial behavior (i.e., be-havior that requires personal sacrifices) with non-kin others dropped across all six societies as children approached middle childhood. However, their rates of prosociality diverged as children began to conform toward the beha-vior of adults in their own societies. The authors claim that their results are consistent with theories that emphasize the importance of acquired cultural norms in shaping choices that require personal sacrifices to assist coopera-tion (House et al., 2013).

It appears that the extent and flexibility of cooperation between groups is predicated by how culturally similar they are. Researchers have claimed that this process, known as "cultural group selection," is possible because cultural variation is structured in populations to a greater degree than genetic vari-ation (Boyd, Richerson, and Henrich, 2011). The premise is that while mi-gration steadily erodes genetic variations between groups, cultural variations between groups are often preserved because migrants adopt the cultural practices of their new group. Such selection acting over human evolutionary history may explain why we cooperate readily with unrelated and unfamiliar individuals and why humans' unprecedented cooperative flexibility may nevertheless be culturally parochial (C. Handley and Mathew, 2020).

Cooperative Brain Processes

Such cooperation seems to be assisted by some hard-wired brain tenden-cies. Social psychologists and social neuroscientists have identified special-ized neural systems that underlie compassion and altruism (Zaki, López, and Mitchell, 2014). Research on the genetic basis of cooperation also appears to demonstrate that social circuitry in the brain has evolved to support cooper-ation among primates and humans (Chang, Gariépy, and Platt, 2013; Reuter et al., 2011). Distinct brain regions have been found to be selectively associ-ated with cooperation and competition, notably the orbitofrontal cortex in cooperation and the inferior parietal and medial prefrontal cortices in com-petition. Cooperation therefore appears to be a socially rewarding process that is associated with specific left medial orbitofrontal cortex involvement (Decety et al., 2004)—that is, cooperation can bring a neural reward to those who operate it or observe it.

Researchers have also looked at what restricts the altruistic mirroring impulse. A non-invasive procedure called theta-burst transcranial magnetic stimulation was used on fifty-eight participants to numb brain activity in specific areas. Participants with numbed-down activity in the prefrontal cortex were found to be 50 percent more generous than participants who were numbed elsewhere in the brain. Subjects who made their decisions very fast about how much to contribute to a common endowment were substantially more generous than subjects who made their decisions slowly. "Forcing subjects to decide quickly increases contributions, whereas instructing them to reflect and forcing them to decide slowly decreases contributions" (Rand, Greene, and Nowak, 2012). In another study, where participants were encouraged to "trust their intuition" when contributing to an endowment, the suggestion increased the sizes of their contributions (Christov-Moore and Iacoboni, 2016). It appears therefore that not only are we are primed to be altruistic and to cooperate but also that our instinct to do so can be dimmed by thinking too much about it!

Genetics Too

Genetics too appears to play a part in shaping tendencies toward helping and cooperation with others. Some people appear to be primed to be more altruistic than others. In a genetics experiment, carriers of at least one genetic allele variation donated about twice as much money as participants without. It was found that those with the OXTR rs53576 G to A variation or AVPR1a RS1/RS3 long to short variation of genes were more likely to exhibit "prosocial" behavior by being more trusting of strangers, contributing more to charitable activities, and participating in more civic duties (Poulin, Holman, and Buffone, 2012).

In another experiment, participants played the dictator game, which economists and other social scientists often use to study decision-making (Kahneman, Knetsch, and Thaler, 1986). In this game, participants are given a certain amount of money to either keep for themselves or share with a stranger. After they have completed the game, researchers compared their payouts with brain scans. Christov-Moore and Iacoboni (2016) found that one-third of the participants who had the strongest responses in the areas of the brain associated with perceiving pain and emotion and imitating others were the most generous: on average, subjects in that group gave away approximately 75 percent of their bounty. This tendency is known as "prosocial resonance" or mirroring impulse, and they believe this impulse to be a primary driving force behind altruism (Christov-Moore and Iacoboni, 2016).

Cooperation Assisted by Norms

According to Bell, Richerson, and McElreath (2009), socially learned behavior and beliefs are much better candidates than genetics to explain the self-sacrificing behavior we often see among strangers, from soldiers who fight for a common good to blood donors who give to strangers (in most of Europe, such donations are voluntary) and people who freely contribute to food banks. While such sharing is normal within groups with whom we share a social identity, sharing beyond our groups appears to be a relatively new value, which has had to be nurtured in that getting people to recognize those in socially new groups as belonging to "our" group is difficult, and it is harder to increase an individual's or group's willingness to share resources as the social distance between the decision maker and the recipient increases (Ma, Pei, and Jin, 2015).

What helped to bind such groups together is thought to be overarching frameworks of belonging, and norms of morality that provided the glue for the necessary expansion of belonging, as groups expanded to survive (Green, 2011). Thus it appears that groups that created social norms that fostered cooperation and were based on a broad societal consensus became more successful and spread farther than others (Fehr and Fischbacher, 2004b). Many of these initial norms were created because of the exigencies of trade. The need for economic institutions that enabled trade to function meant that these were the first national and international institutions to thrive. Markets often had sets of regulations and behaviors that broke down social barriers, enforced fairness between traders, and curtailed attempts to control trade for one's own benefit (Blanton, 2016). Functioning markets thus became a stimulator for the creation of institutions that enabled strangers to cooperate and to rely on each other (Bowles and Gintis, 2011). Eventually, the markets also required legal, policy, business, and economic institutions to remain sustainable. These increased the ease of cooperation, and, in some cases, developed mechanisms to punish those who refused to cooperate (Burnham and Johnson, 2005).

Moral frameworks that were enforced by systems of sanctions and rewards also increased the reproductive success of individuals who functioned well in such environments, as well as the development of social emotions like empathy and social shame that assisted cooperation (Boyd and Richerson, 2009). Such larger identities were also helped by the development of group identity markers such as language, religion, and nationality. Over time, community leaders gradually discovered how to strengthen shared identity via the strategic use of group symbolism, such as history, flags, parades, and national anthems. Group identity norms and culture thus provided a solution to the need to extend one's group partnerships to larger groups. Because cultural evolution can happen at a faster rate than genetic evolution, it allowed humans to adapt quickly to complex, variable environments (Boyd and Richerson, 1985).

Punishment

Important as they are, cultural, legal, and economic norms are not always sufficient to curb an individual's, group's, or nation's tendencies to act for their own benefit. Agreement on norms often requires the sanction of punishment to ensure that people will sacrifice for their group. There is a need to manage "free riders" (i.e., those who refuse to cooperate but nevertheless try to benefit from some good without expending effort or paying for it; Fischbacher, Gächter, and Fehr, 2001; Stallen and Sanfey, 2013). One of the most consistent findings across studies on the neural mechanisms of cooperation (Fehr and Gächter, 2000) has been that the addition of a punishment option to the public goods game—a standard test of experimental economics—considerably increased cooperation levels (until there was almost 100 percent cooperation), and in the absence of such an option, cooperation levels dropped (Dong, Zhang, and Tao, 2016).

Such has always been the tension between individual and group gains. Social selection mechanisms such as exclusion from the marriage market, denial of the fruits of cooperative activities, banishment, and execution would have exerted strong selection against genes tending toward antisocial behavior. Social selection in favor of genes that predisposed individuals toward prosociality are also easy to imagine (Bell et al., 2009).

The existence of punishments by third parties for norm violations enabled the rapid development of agreed social norms and the evolution of cooperation among group members (Rand et al., 2009).

An important caveat, however, is that researchers have also found that social exclusion decreases the likelihood of future prosocial behavior occurring (Twenge et al., 2007). It appears that having been socially excluded—for example, in prison—can cause prosocial behavior to drop significantly, and this can have significant consequences for punishments such as criminalization and sanctions.

Role of Leadership

Almost all collaboration requires leadership, and it appears that our seemingly unreasonable devotion to some leaders may have developed to facilitate such cooperation in large groups (see Chapter 6 of this volume). According to evolutionary theory, "charisma" in a leader is the ability to convince followers that you can get the members of a wide group to cooperate. "Charismatic leadership and followership is a dynamic process in which leaders signal their ability to benefit the group by increasing the perceived likelihood that cooperation will succeed" (Grabo and van Vugt, 2016). Leaders therefore have always been crucial in enabling cooperation among their people and in eliciting cooperation with others beyond their own group. Unfortunately, as has been noted in Chapter 6 of this book, today's leaders are mostly still transactional leaders and are often more concerned with cooperation within their group, and with local and national leadership, than with the requirements of global leadership—that is, the type of leadership that would seem to be the major requirement for the earth's future.

The Future

That we live in a radically interconnected world has become a truism. Indeed, this age of internationalism and the Internet might well be called the age of inter: there is nothing that is not interconnected, interdependent, interwoven, interlaced, interactive, or interfacing with something else to make it what it is. (McMahan, 2009, p. 131)

Robert Wright's iconic book *Nonzero* (Wright, 1999) showed how he thought history would gradually weave us into ever-vaster webs of interdependence. It is true that institutions of regional and global interdependence, based on shared economic, technological, market, legal, fuel, environmental, and political networks, are increasingly the norm and have proliferated in the two decades since Wright wrote his book. It is hard to imagine that the world can retreat from such interdependence without nations harming themselves and each other and destroying the common good that is the earth. The stock markets are now all global and react to events in an interdependent way. World trade is increasingly global, with most goods—particularly food and technical goods—depending increasingly on worldwide networks for their production and distribution. As I write, the Covid-19 virus is rampaging across the world: like environmental concerns, it is a worldwide challenge that cannot be dealt with solely on a national basis. It appears that half of the ventilators used in acute hospitals worldwide, which are essential to the treatment of Covid-19 illness, are currently manufactured in Ireland (IDA Ireland, 2020), and half the world's necessary masks to protect from the infection were made in China before the coronavirus emerged there (Bradsher and Alderman, 2020).

In addition, and of particular relevance for the peacebuilder, almost all conflicts today are becoming ever more complex by the addition of proxy and shadow partners, by the ubiquitous global sources of weapons, and by the increasingly problematic power of social media (see Chapter 8 of this volume). The social scientist Steven Pinker argues in his book *The Better Angels of Our Nature* that war and violent conflict have been declining steadily, and he hopes they may soon be obsolete (Pinker, 2012). Pinker believes that evolutionary forces have shaped human nature into a complex amalgam of the best and worst of our characteristics. Yet he argues that even while we retain our many conflictual and violent impulses, historical trends such as stronger governments; increased prosperity, literacy, education, and trade; and the empowerment of women are allowing us to effectively tame many of them.

However, looking at the world today, it appears that our human hardwiring and cultural wiring have not yet caught up with what is needed for today's interdependence challenges—maintaining a healthy environment, large-scale migration, pandemics, etc.—and the need to develop institutions that can match such challenges. While this book, and its many noted resources, may have been unsettling in unearthing the particular tendencies of human beings that make conflict and war so easy to develop, it is reassuring to know that as human beings we have in the past faced many conflicted and cooperative challenges, and as a human race we have survived such challenges and thrived by increasing our willingness to share information and resources and help with others beyond our tribe. Hopefully, by better understanding the often unconscious legacies of our human evolutionary development, which are the subject of this book, we may better address them and more powerfully elicit the tendencies of altruism and cooperation that will be needed in our increasingly interdependent world in the decades ahead.

10

Peacebuilding More Successfully?

Keep Watching Out for New Knowledge!

As you will have noticed, much of what is in this book has come from relatively new sciences—political psychology, neuroscience, biopsychology, biopsychology, genopolitics, political physiology, behavioral genetics, cognitive neuroscience, etc.—many of which are still at the early stages of their development. Many of their findings are still tentative and leave plenty of room for newer and more certain knowledge to emerge over the coming decades. So please keep an eye out for what knowledge is yet to come.

In the meantime, the following are some ideas drawn from the insights in the book, and the work of the many peacebuilding institutions to keep in mind as you set about your peacebuilding task. They are listed in no particular order.

Do not base strategies solely—or even primarily—on reason. Conflicts are usually fraught with unstated instincts and emotions, which, unless addressed, will remain as barriers to successful peacebuilding. Remember, for change to happen, groups, nations, leaders, and people need to be both emotionally *and* rationally engaged in peacebuilding.

Remember that anger and aggression often come from fear. Fear is usually hidden behind anger. Hence it is useful to ask ourselves and others about what people/communities/nations are afraid of, rather than what just they are angry about. Better understanding the feelings behind their arguments, and what their individual and collective amygdalae are telling them, may suggest different approaches that may be more productive.

Try to ensure societies in which people can behave at their best, not their worst. Remember that most of us are a mixture of both good and bad, and contexts often define our behavior. It is therefore important to help develop environments that are helpful in enabling people to live peacefully together. It is now well established that contexts of, for example, horizontal inequalities (Stewart, 2008), where people are excluded or mistreated because of their identity, are one of the most likely causes of most conflicts today.

Our Brains at War. Mari Fitzduff, Oxford University Press (2021). © Oxford University Press.
DOI: 10.1093/oso/9780197512654.003.0011

Peacebuilding therefore must address, or promise to address, such contexts, if it is to be sustainable. As noted by Pinker (2012), the more successful we are at creating effective political and legal institutions, and the safer our societies become, the less we are likely to kill each other.

Don't bother (too much) with "fact"-checking. Recognize that rational argument has its limits. To logically attack the opinions of someone who has a heartfelt belief that is socially shared with many others in their network is not often a useful strategy. Focusing on fact-checking is often ineffectual, as seeming "errors" often exist because they serve a social or psychological need on the part of an individual or group. Thus the "truths" felt at, for example, Trump rallies will matter far more to his supporters than those expounded in newspapers, by other politicians, or by academics.

Remember, we are, all of us, far less rational than we think. As peacebuilders we too bring many of our natural social instincts and biases to bear on our work. Checking these, by partnering with people who have a different emotional and cognitive temperament, a different cultural background, and differing perspectives on peacebuilding needs can be useful. Helping other people (and ourselves) to understand their (and our) own, often unconscious, feelings of bias is also important. Hidden biases can be elicited easily from almost everyone using dialogue techniques that are designed to do this (Fitzduff and Williams, 2019). Having to face up to and own one's biases is a humbling process, but it can lead to more openness in understanding such biases in others and more success in trying to address them.

We all divide the world into "us" and "them"—and we usually support "us". People should not be surprised that all of us, even peacebuilders, may at times have negative feelings toward other groups. Such personal and group feelings are often a remnant of our family, community, and national warning systems about those who are seen as "strangers." However, it is important to note that while we may not be responsible for their existence, it is what we do as a result of such feelings is what is important.

Remember that people usually do "believe" what they say. Our opponents are not necessarily uninformed or unintelligent but rather, at a very basic level, they experience different emotional and cognitive frameworks and thus interpret the world differently. So while people may stubbornly resist factual evidence about issues such as their history and behavior, the sovereignty of a region, their need to occupy particular territory, their perspective on climate change, the appropriate behavior for a president, etc., it is often more helpful to see such viewpoints as coming from emotions that are often unspecified. Eliciting these—sensitively, of course—can help toward exploring alternative ways of dealing with the conflicts under discussion.

When faced with a moral difference, be careful of your own instincts. Groups/tribes/nations often have distinctive moral and/or religious commitments that others may not recognize as authoritative. However, we should all remember that things that seem morally obvious to us now were not necessarily so in the past. So, before we assert certainties in relation to others' morality, we should note how often ours have changed and how some moral certainties that seemed invincible to us are no longer so. Attitudes to homosexuality, capital punishment, "just" wars, abortion, meat-eating, women's inferiority, female circumcision, etc. have significantly changed what may once have seemed to be immutable truths for many of us. So keeping an open mind and avoiding certainties on our own part is a useful skill for peacebuilders.

Remember—most people are conservative, for very good reasons. Change takes time, and more time. Conservatism/traditionalism is more normal than liberalism. Groups throughout history have been driven by those whose intentions are to "conserve" what societal arrangements have worked in their past. Conservatives are usually the majority in any society. People's and groups' reasons for not changing are often "rational" when understood within their own framework, if not in yours. So while it often makes sense in the first place to work on agreements with those who seem better able to handle uncertainty and dialogue with out-groups, remember that peacebuilding processes have to eventually include the conservative majority.

Find out who matters to the people or groups you are working with. People, communities, and nations can more easily face change when they trust the sources who are suggesting it. Close friends, family members, beer buddies, or trusted religious, business, or community leaders often work better to emotionally (and occasionally rationally) influence people when facts and experts do not. This may mean enlisting leaders who are aligned in some ways to those who are most resistant to change to acquire their help with any needed change strategies.

Use "norm entrepreneurs" to sell change. Creating new norms in a society is likely to be a more fruitful pathway for changing behaviors than a process targeted at changing personal beliefs in the first place. Such change can be helped by using "norm entrepreneurs" (Sunstein, 1996)—that is, people who can suggest a new or amended norm for social change and who are trusted by communities and nations (Mickiewicz and Rebmann, 2020). Such norm entrepreneurs can reduce the perceived emotional cost of societal change for communities, as well as suggest the benefits of such change.

Create institutions that promote familiarity with "others." Fears are often (not always!) based on ignorance. The more that people and groups intermingle and work together on common issues over a sustained period of time, the less likely they are to stereotype each other. Increased exposure to other identities helps to suppress the "other" bias within the brain circuitry. Schools, universities, workplaces, youth groups, sports groups, and civil service and government groups, as well as cultural and religious institutions, can all play an important part in decreasing feelings of suspicion between groups. Such institutions can help normalize cross-cutting engagement by people from all colors and creeds and diminish the cross-group anxieties that are normally present when such cooperation is rare. Note, however, that no matter how much intermingling happens, a continuance of inequities and exclusion between groups will diminish the trust between them.

Develop new groups for people to belong to. People need to belong somewhere. It makes it easier for them to adjust to change if there are social and political institutions that are open to people who are willing to change their perspective, attitudes, and behaviors. Without such new or reformed groups or institutions to belong to, new perceptions and behaviors can quickly die in the face of personal, community, and group isolation, which can make it easier for people to return to older prejudices and loyalties.

Take care to note differing cultural processes. There are many ways in which cultures differ in terms of how people relate to each other. Being aware of how societies order themselves in terms of, for example, their level of deference to authority, the importance of reputation in a high-context culture, the norms of the how and the why of criticisms, the nuances of eye contact and personal space, and the sensitivities of gender differences can assist in developing more appropriate and more effective strategies for peacebuilding.

Ceasefires matter. A respite from ongoing daily violence through ceasefires can be very important in providing some emotional space for people to think about the future. Despite negative reactions to such when they are mooted or happen—cynicism, disbelief, "it's only winning time for the other side to regroup," etc.—ceasefires can allow societies' amygdalae to relax just a little and let more long-term rational and institutional factors come to the table in the search for an agreement.

Sell peace agreements to the heart and not just the head. Peace agreements are often felt as lose–lose agreements because of the compromises both sides have had to make. Agreements therefore often fall apart because although the cognitive skills of those involved may have crafted clever political and social compromises, constituents fail to feel emotionally that they are gaining. Peace agreements should be sold through trusted people and groups and the media to elicit feelings of hope and possibility. The gains of such agreements should also be notable from an early stage to ensure continued emotional hope in the possibility of sustained peace.

Note that the advent of peace is not an emotional gain for everyone. Many people will have found exciting and meaningful roles for themselves and their groups in their war-related activities. Without opportunities for continuing to use their energies and adopt new roles in a way that excludes illegal violence, a post-conflict society is likely to be more fragile and less sustainable.

Remember to work with diasporas. Because of the often insecure nature of their membership of a national or regional group and the need to prove themselves loyal to a cause, diaspora communities are often the last to be open to the compromises necessary for peacebuilding. This can delay a peace agreement unless prior work is done with them on the necessity for such peacebuilding. Finding new ways to take forward their need to continue to belong to an identity group while also moving ahead with any necessary political and social changes is in many cases important if peacebuilding is to be sustainable.

Use traditionalmedia to help change social norms. There are many ways in which traditional media can assist in developing emotional readiness for peacebuilding. Sensitively handled discussions on the media about possible peace agreements can accustom people to hearing about possible compromises, so that their amygdalae are not continually alert for possible losses from such agreements. Radio soap operas can help people understand the needs and beliefs of differing communities and increase the empathy factor between them (Paluck and Green, 2009). Peace journalists and others can attempt to take on board and talk about the diverse views that exist in a conflict, and traditional newspapers can carry articles with, for example, another group's point of view (Youngblood, 2017).

Use the law—where it will be obeyed. Law can be the ultimate behavior changer in situations where legal institutions exist and are trusted and obeyed (Lessig, 1995). If a government is trusted (enough!), legal changes can be very effective in creating behavioral changes. This is because people in a situation of cognitive or emotional dissonance (Festinger, 1962) will usually adjust their emotions to such changes even if they were hostile to them in the first place—for example, laws about smoking, seat belts, and motorcycle helmets, as well as laws particularly relevant to peacebuilding such as anti-discrimination, equal opportunity, and hate crime laws. The implementation of such laws can be helped by publicity programs that can sway people's emotions toward the required legislation.

Young men in particular need positive "heroic" opportunities. Young men, who are the main perpetrators and the main victims in all conflicts, need opportunities to use their biopsychological energies and tendencies for either better or worse purposes. Curbing their attraction to joining illegal violent groups often requires creating alternative and positive opportunities for their energies and their ideals through, for example, employment, civil society action, or marriage and children (Hoffman, 2001). It also means minimizing the inequities and exclusion that they may feel, which are often used to justify their violence. Also, given the attraction for some men in the offers of available sex and female relationships through joining a jihad group, addressing the secretive and repressive approach to sexuality in many Middle Eastern countries through modern sex education may help to manage this pull factor to extremist groups for young men.

Provide modern values and sex education where it can be done. There is an obvious attraction for some men in the offers of available sex and female relationships through joining a jihad group, and this is often used as part of a recruitment drive. Addressing the secretive and repressive approach to sexuality in many Middle Eastern countries through modern sex education may help to manage this pull factor to extremist groups for young men.

Help leaders who want to become more inclusive. Leaders will often say they cannot move ahead of their people lest they lose votes or support. Finding ways to reassure them that they can be more inclusive in their concerns will depend on the possibilities that exist for changing the views of enough of their followers. Peace polls such as those by Irwin (2006) are deemed to have helped intransigent politicians move their positions by showing them that their constituents will move somewhat faster than the politicians think. Another project is its Shared Society Project of the Club of Madrid,[1] which is composed of former prime ministers and presidents who

---

[1] http://www.clubmadrid.org/programa/shared-societies-project/

are available to work on a peer-to-peer basis with current leaders on creating more inclusive societies.

New leadership? Assisting the development of a new, more inclusive generation of leaders through community activities/local development/national and international training programs can be helpful. This is particularly true when such programs are carried out on a cross-community/national basis and provide plenty of time to develop empathy and trust between the leaders and groups.

Build trust in relevant peacebuilding institutions. Building cross-community institutions that are trusted by people and that have a role in developing inclusive and equitable societies can be helpful, even without the open support of opposing leaders and politicians. Such institutions can prepare a society to believe that fairness and inclusion is possible and thus make it easier for eventual peace agreements to be made (Fitzduff, 2016).

Involve more women peacebuilders. Women are often lacking in senior roles in peace processes despite the evidence that women's participation in conflict prevention and resolution can improve outcomes before, during, and after conflict. Without their participation, peace agreements are 64 percent likely to fail. There is evidence that women's capacity for empathy is greater than that of men, and their gender and size are less likely to threaten male participants, which can provide extra mediation opportunities. Including more women in senior roles in peacebuilding processes therefore provides extra dividends in such processes (N-Peace Network, 2009).

Develop cyber-warfare peacebuilding skills. Many future wars will be won or lost through the use of social media. There is an urgent need for peacebuilders to develop resources that can limit or counteract the destructive emotional effect of social media on peacebuilding processes. According to Mercy Corps (2019), these processes include influencing policies and regulations of governments, multinational bodies, industry associations, and technology companies to develop and fund moderators who can assess and challenge propaganda aimed at sowing confusion or hatred between groups and nations. Information literacy programs are also increasingly important in today's world. The Baltic States have digital literacy campaigns to enable their citizens to better navigate a world of "likes" and "dislikes" and to distinguish lies and half-truths from facts (Zoria, 1018). Estonia has created a

Cyber Defence Unit (Kaska, Osula, and Stinissen, 2013), which consists of an army of volunteer specialists in information technology who focus on international cyber-defense activities. Civil society peacebuilders such as the Alliance for Peacebuilding, through their Technology and Social Media platform are also harnessing their capacities to counter destructive social media processes that are increasingly making their peacebuilding work more difficult (https://www.allianceforpeacebuilding.org/technology-and-social-media-wg). But much more needs to be done urgently to counteract the damage being done to peacebuilding through the negative process of social media.

Suggestions for Peacebuilding Dialogue Work

Where dialogue processes are to take place between politicians, militia leaders, civil society peacebuilders, etc., the following suggestions can help to make them a success.

Perspective training. The power of increasing empathy and cooperation through perspective-shifting—that is, changing the way people understand and think about other groups, has been examined using functional magnetic imaging (Bruneau and Saxe, 2012). It shows that encouraging perspective-shifting through meeting and talking can, if done effectively, actually alter the neural circuits concerned with identity differences, encouraging groups to increase their prosocial behavior toward each other. However, such sharing cannot ignore histories of perceived inequalities, or its effect will be temporary and limited.

Increase oxytocin during conflicted groups encounters. Accounts from peacebuilders about how peace agreements were eventually reached often point to informal and unrecognized personal and group processes that appear to have been successful in increasing oxytocin and trust levels. Such processes can be increased by gestures such as gift-giving, meal-sharing, alcohol where it is culturally permitted (just a modicum—too much can make us belligerent!), positive physical gestures, expressions of understanding and appreciation, sharing of family stories, and group singing. Facilitators and mediators should provide plenty of space for such personal encounters to happen informally as well as formally.

Deal constructively with the past. Collective memories of the past need to be reviewed and teased out together with opposing groups so that the differences in remembering can be shared, and the feelings (as opposed to just the "facts" each group remembers) behind such memories can be understood. While one can argue with another person's facts, one cannot argue with their feelings.

Do single identity work. Bringing together groups without single identity work (i.e., discussion within identity communities about issues on which the people in the group differ) can be counterproductive. If groups have not had a chance to deal with their own differences, they are likely to assume a narrower collective stance about their beliefs and objectives in order not to stray from norms of group loyalty (Church et al., 2002).

Encourage moderates to speak first in group work. The first person to speak in an intergroup process will usually set the emotional tone of the dialogues that follow. Therefore encouraging group moderates to speak first in an intergroup process can help relieve concerns about betrayal on the part of participants who are fearful of being seen as outliers in their group.

Increasing cognitive complexity. One program openly addressing the need for integrative complexity is the Sabaoon rehabilitation program for violent extremists in Pakistan. This uses an innovative model rooted in sociology and psychology that seeks to increase the students' integrative complexity to decrease "black and white" thinking and improve critical thinking (Peracha, Khan, and Savage, 2012). Also, resilience training aimed at longitudinal increases in self-esteem, agency, and empathy in Muslim immigrant youths resulted in negative attitudes toward ideology-based violence on the part of the participants (Feddes, Mann, and Doosje, 2015).

More effective talking. For dialogue work between groups to be effective, a number of conditions are useful to keep in mind. The contact must foster relatively equal status between the two groups, and contact must be frequent and must help close enough trust relationships to be derived from these interactions. It is also useful if the contact entails working toward a common goal on some issue that requires sustained cooperation between the groups. Such dialogue work will be less effective in changing a conflict context if it does not also effectively change the social and political context of the particular conflict. Therefore, the work is often of no avail unless it can also include political, military, or community leaders who can get to know and trust one another sufficiently to energize political agreements.

Conclusions

Remember, we are predisposed, not predestined. While personal biological factors such as brain architecture, hormones, and genetic heritage are important, they do not by themselves cause a behavior by regulating it so much as by sensitizing it to particular environments. Changing those environments can (somewhat) change our attitudinal and behavioral tendencies.

We are all born with different tendencies. We are born with different tendencies toward fear, diversity, novelty, risk-taking, and change, and these tendencies will have significant consequences for many of our social attitudes to out-groups and security issues. However, our brains and our attitudes can coevolve if we have enough societal security, enough exposure to others who think differently, and a context that stimulates emotional and cognitive reflections on tendencies and biases that are different from our own. Nevertheless, we also need to remember that for some time after fear has apparently somewhat diminished, contexts of danger can easily return us to our previous personal and community tendencies and biases.

Believe that individual and social change is possible. Apart from a very small number of the mentally ill (i.e., psychopaths and sociopaths who do not feel empathy for others nor guilt about harming others), people and communities can and do change when the conditions are right for more empathy and inclusiveness for traditional "others." All our histories tell of people who at one period in their lives freely injured and killed people from other groups, who eventually become productive members of societies. Our histories also tell us of nations that have moved beyond their wars to trade and partner with those who had been traditional enemies. Updating and invigorating our beliefs in the possibility of change can determine how we help our world move forward.

Building a larger "we"? The human race has come a long way from where we started. Our various genetic and physical tendencies have been powerful in enabling us (mostly) to live together relatively peacefully and to survive as communities. Such tendencies have helped us to create a sophisticated network of communities who are now globally interdependent on matters of trade and communication, although rather less so on many social attitudes and behaviors. Many challenges remain: environmental challenges, growing resource inequalities, proxy wars, and, above all, the challenge of psyches that have been bred to thrive within smaller communities than those that are emerging today.

It is useful to remember that as humans we have been left with many instincts and feelings that served our ancestors well when their environments were very different. Despite this, in a relatively short time the world in which we live has become an interconnected and dynamic space where our ability to collaborate rather than compete has been vital for its social and economic success. Understanding the worst in human tendencies and how easy they are to evoke in most of us is crucial. However, no less crucial is the knowledge that our history has proved to us, as ever-evolving human beings, that we can move beyond our current tribes to interact with others to ensure that we expand the sum of human good for all in this tiny, interconnected world.

References

Acharya, S. and Shukla, S. (2012) Mirror neurons: Enigma of the metaphysical modular brain. *Journal of Natural Science, Biology and Medicine*, 3(2), 118–124.

Achenbach, J. (2015, March) Why do many reasonable people doubt science? *National Geographic*.

Adams, S. (2015, August 26) Do your testosterone and cortisol levels dictate your leadership ability? *Forbes*. https://www.forbes.com/sites/susanadams/2015/08/26/do-your-testosterone-and-cortisol-levels-dictate-your-leadership-ability/#655ea12c7dbb

Agara, T. (2015) Gendering terrorism: Women, gender, terrorism and suicide bombers. *International Journal of Humanities and Social Science*, 5(6/1), 115–125.

Agiesta, J. (2015) Misperceptions persist about Obama's faith, but aren't so widespread. *CNN*. https://edition.cnn.com/2015/09/13/politics/barack-obama-religion-christian-misperceptions/index.html

Albarello, F., Foroni, F., Hewstone, M., and Rubini, M. (2017) "They are all alike": When negative minority outgroups are generalized onto superordinate inclusive outgroups. *International Journal of Intercultural Relations*, 73, 59–73.

Alford, J.R., Funk, C.L., and Hibbing, J.R. (2005) Are political orientations genetically transmitted? *American Political Science Review*, 99(2), 153–167.

Alison, M. (2003) Cogs in the wheel? Women in the Liberation Tigers of Tamil Eelam. *Civil Wars*, 6(4), 37–54.

Allard, E.S. and Kensinger, E.A. (2014, April 10) Age-related differences in neural recruitment during the use of cognitive reappraisal and selective attention as emotion regulation strategies. *Frontiers in Psychology*. https://doi.org/10.3389/fpsyg.2014.00296

Allen, J. (2008, September 10) No consensus on who was behind Sept 11: Global poll. *Reuters*. https://www.reuters.com/article/us-sept11-qaeda-poll/no-consensus-on-who-was-behind-sept-11-global-poll-idUSN1035876620080910

Al-Rodham, N. (2013) The future of international relations: A symbiotic realism theory. *BBVA OpenMind*. https://www.bbvaopenmind.com/en/articles/the-future-of-international-relations/

Al-Rodham, N. (2014, February 27) The neurochemistry of power has implications for political change. *OXPOL: The Oxford University Politics Blog*. https://blog.politics.ox.ac.uk/neurochemistry-power-implications-political-change/

Al-Zawahiri, A. (2005) Letter from al-Zawahiri to al-Zarqawi. *Federation of American Scientists*. https://fas.org/irp/news/2005/10/letter_in_english.pdf

Ambady, N. (2011) The mind in the world: Culture and the brain. *Association for Psychological Science*. https://www.psychologicalscience.org/observer/the-mind-in-the-world-culture-and-the-brain

Ames, D.L. and Fiske, S.T. (2010) Cultural neuroscience. *Asian Journal of Social Psychology*, 13(2), 72–82.

Amodio, D.M. (2014) The neuroscience of prejudice and stereotyping. *Nature Reviews Neuroscience*, 15(10), 670–682.

Amodio, D.M., Devine, P.G., and Harmon-Jones, E. (2008) Individual differences in the regulation of intergroup bias: The role of conflict monitoring and neural signals for control. *Journal of Personality and Social Psychology*, 94(1), 60–74.

Amodio, D.M. and Frith, C.D. (2006) Meeting of minds: The medial frontal cortex and social cognition. *Nature Reviews Neuroscience*, 7(4), 268–277.

Amodio, D.M., Jost, J.T., Master, S.L., and Yee, C.M. (2007) Neurocognitive correlates of liberalism and conservatism. *Nature Neuroscience*, 10(10), 1246–1247.

Analysis: Islamic State media output goes into sharp decline (2017, November 23) *BBC Monitoring*. https://monitoring.bbc.co.uk/product/c1dnnj2k

Anderson, J. (2017, January 31) The psychology of why 94 deaths from terrorism are scarier than 301,797 deaths from guns. *Quartz*. https://qz.com/898207/the-psychology-of-why-americans-are-more-scared-of-terrorism-than-guns-though-guns-are-3210-times-likelier-to-kill-them/

Angier, N. (2012, April) Edward O. Wilson's new take on human nature. *Smithsonian Magazine*. https://www.smithsonianmag.com/science-nature/edward-o-wilsons-new-take-on-human-nature-160810520/

Antonakis, J. and Dalgas, O. 2009. Predicting elections: Child's play! *Science*, 323(5918), 1183.

Apicella, C.L. and Silk, J.B. (2019) The evolution of human cooperation. *Current Biology*, 29(11), R447–R450.

Appiah, K.A. (2018) *The lies that bind: Rethinking identity*. New York: Liveright.

Arendt, H. (1963) *Eichmann in Jerusalem: A report on the banality of evil*. London: Viking Press.

Arvey, R., Rotundo, M., Johnson, W., Zhang, Z., and McGue, M. (2006) The determinants of leadership role occupancy: Genetic and personality factors. *Leadership Quarterly*, 17(1), 1–20.

Asghar, R. (2016, February 26) The science behind Donald Trump's appeal. *Forbes*. https://www.forbes.com/sites/robasghar/2016/02/26/donald-trumps-messy-leadership-lesson-alpha-dogs-still-have-bite/

Aslam, S. (2020, February 10) Twitter by the numbers: Stats, demographics & fun facts. *Omnicore*. https://www.omnicoreagency.com/twitter-statistics/

Asp, E.W., Ramchandran, K., and Tranel, D. (2012) Authoritarianism, religious fundamentalism, and the human prefrontal cortex. *Neuropsychology*, 26(4), 414–421.

Atran, S. (2015, November 15) Mindless terrorists? The truth about Isis is much worse. *The Guardian*.

Atran, S., Axelrod, R., and Davis, R. (2007) Sacred barriers to conflict resolution. *Science*, 317(5841), 1039–1040.

Atran, S., Sheikh, H., and Gómez, Á. (2014) Devoted actors fight for close comrades and sacred cause. *Proceedings of the National Academy of Sciences of the United States of America*, 111(50), 17702–17703.

Bakker, E. and de Graaf, B. (2010) Lone wolves: How to prevent this phenomenon? *International Centre for Counter-Terrorism*. https://www.icct.nl/download/file/ICCT-Bakker-deGraaf-EM-Paper-Lone-Wolves.pdf

Balthazard, P.A., Waldman, D.A., Thatcher, R.W., and Hannah, S.T. (2012) Differentiating transformational and nontransformational leaders on the basis of neurological imaging. *Leadership Quarterly*, 23, 244–258.

Banks, C. (2019) Introduction: Women, gender, and terrorism: Gendering terrorism. *Women & Criminal Justice*, 29, 181–187.

Banks, S.J., Eddy, K.T., Angstadt, M., Nathan, P.J., and Phan, K.L. (2007) Amygdala–frontal connectivity during emotion regulation. *Social Cognitive and Affective Neuroscience*, 2(4), 303–312.

Bar-Tal, D., Chernyak-Hai, L., Schori, N., and Gundar, A. (2009) A sense of self-perceived collective victimhood in intractable conflicts. *International Review of the Red Cross*, 91(874), 229–258.

Battaglia, F.P., Benchenane, K., Sirota, A., Pennartz, C.M., and Wiener, S.I. (2011) The hippocampus: Hub of brain network communication for memory. *Trends in Cognitive Science*, 15(7), 310–318.

Beauregard, M., Lévesque, J., and Bourgouin, P. (2001) Neural correlates of conscious self-regulation of emotion. *Journal of Neuroscience*, 21(18), RC165.

Belasen, A.T. (2015) Deception and failure: Mitigating leader-centric behaviours. In A.T. Belasen and R. Toma (eds.), *Confronting corruption in business: Trusted leadership, civic engagement* (pp. 183–216). New York: Routledge,

Belief in God and prejudice reduced by directing magnetic energy into the brain. (2015, October 14) *Science Daily*. https://www.sciencedaily.com/releases/2015/10/151014084955.htm

Bell, A.V., Richerson, P.J., and McElreath, R. (2009) Culture rather than genes provides greater scope for the evolution of large-scale human prosociality. *Proceedings of the National Academy of Sciences of the United States of America*, 106(42), 17671–17674.

Benedict, H. (2008, August 13) Why soldiers rape: Culture of misogyny, illegal occupation, fuel sexual violence in military. *In These Times*. http://inthesetimes.com/article/3848

Benmelech, E. and Berrebi, C. (2007) Human capital and the productivity of suicide bombers. *Journal of Economic Perspectives*, 21(3), 223–238.

Ben-Ze'ev, E., Ginio, R., and Winter, J. (eds.) (2010) *Shadows of war: A social history of silence in the twentieth century*. Cambridge: Cambridge University Press.

Bergen, P. (2016, June 14) Why do terrorists commit terrorism? *New York Times*.

Bergland, C. (2012, December 25) The evolutionary biology of altruism. *Psychology Today*. https://www.psychologytoday.com/blog/the-athletes-way/201212/the-evolutionary-biology-altruism

Berlatsky, N. (2014, December 11) The neuroscience of altruism. *Pacific Standard*. https://psmag.com/social-justice/neuroscience-altruism-donald-pfaff-brain-morality-96067

Bernhardt, B.C. and Singer, T. (2012) The neural basis of empathy. *Annual Review of Neuroscience*, 35, 1–23.

Berns, G., Bell, E., Capra, C.M., Prietula, M.J., Moore, S., Anderson, B., Ginges, J., and Atran, S. (2012) The price of your soul: Neural evidence for the non-utilitarian representation of sacred values. *Philosophical Transactions of the Royal Society of London. Series B, Biological Sciences*, 367(1589), 754–762.

Berridge, K.C. and Kringelbach, M.L. (2015) Pleasure systems in the brain. *Neuron*, 86(3), 646–664.

Bigio, J. and Turkington, R. (2019, March 27) U.S. counterterrorism's big blindspot: Women. *New Republic*. https://newrepublic.com/article/153402/us-counterterrorisms-big-blindspot-women

Bjorklund, D.F. (2006) Mother knows best: Epigenetic inheritance, maternal eVects, and the evolution of human intelligence. *Developmental Review*, 26(2), 213–224.

Blanton, R.E. with Fargher, L.F. (2016) *How humans cooperate: Confronting the challenges of collective action*. Boulder: University Press of Colorado.

Bloom, P. (2013) *Just babies: The origins of good and evil.* New York: Crown.

Bobula, K.A. (2011) *This is your brain on bias . . . or, the neuroscience of bias.* Faculty Lecture Series. Vancouver, WA: Clark College.

Böckler, A., Tusche, A., Schmidt, P., and Singer, T. (2018) Distinct mental trainings differentially affect altruistically motivated, norm motivated, and self-reported pro-social behaviour. *Scientific Reports,* 8(13560). https://www.nature.com/articles/s41598-018-31813-8

Bonanno, G.A. and Jost, J.T. (2006) Conservative shift among high-exposure survivors of the September 11th terrorist attacks. *Basic and Applied Social Psychology,* 28(4), 311–323.

Booth, R. (2014, June 30) Facebook reveals news feed experiment to control emotions. *The Guardian.* https://www.theguardian.com/technology/2014/jun/29/facebook-users-emotions-news-feeds

Bordin, J. (2011) A crisis of trust and cultural incompatibility: A Red Team study of mutual perceptions of Afghan national security force personnel and U.S. soldiers in understanding and mitigating the phenomena of ANSF-committed fratricide-murders. *The National Security Archive, George Washington University.* https://nsarchive2.gwu.edu/NSAEBB/NSAEBB370/docs/Document%2011.pdf

Botha, A. and Abdile, M. (2014) *Radicalisation and al-Shabaab recruitment in Somalia.* Pretoria: Institute for Security Studies.

Boutin, C. (2006, August 22) Snap judgments decide a face's character, psychologist finds. *Princeton University.* https://www.princeton.edu/news/2006/08/22/snap-judgments-decide-faces-character-psychologist-finds

Bowles, S. and Gintis, H. (2011) *A cooperative species: Human reciprocity and its evolution.* Princeton, NJ: Princeton University Press.

Boyd, R. and Richerson, P. (1985) *Culture and the evolutionary process.* Chicago: University of Chicago Press.

Boyd, R. and Richerson, P. (2009) Culture and the evolution of human cooperation. *Philosophical Transactions of the Royal Society B: Biological Sciences,* 364(1533). https://doi.org/10.1098/rstb.2009.0134

Boyd, R., Richerson, P., and Henrich, J. (2011) Rapid cultural adaptation can facilitate the evolution of large-scale cooperation. *Behavioral Ecology and Sociobiology,* 65(3), 431–444.

Bradsher, K. and Alderman, S. (2020, March 13) The world needs masks: China makes them, but has been hoarding them. *New York Times.* https://www.nytimes.com/2020/03/13/business/masks-china-coronavirus.html

Bridge, D.J. and Voss, J.L. (2014) Hippocampal binding of novel information with dominant memory traces can support both memory stability and change. *Journal of Neuroscience,* 34(6), 2203–2213.

Bridgeman, B. (2003) *Psychology and evolution: The origins of mind.* Thousand Oaks, CA: SAGE.

Brigham, J.C., Bennett, L.B., Meissner, C., and Mitchell, T. (2007) The influence of race on eyewitness memory. In R.C. Lindsay, D. Ross, J.D. Read, and M. Toglia (eds.), *Handbook of eyewitness psychology:* Vol. 2, *Memory for people* (pp. 257–281). Mahwah, NJ: Erlbaum.

Brody, G.H. and Stoneman, Z. (1985) Peer imitation: An examination of status and competence hypotheses. *Journal of Genetic Psychology,* 146(2), 161–170.

Bronner, G. (2015) Terrorism and rationality. In G. Manzo (ed.), *Theories and social mechanisms: Essays in honour of Mohamed Cherkaoui* (p. 858). Oxford: Bardwell Press.

Brown, A.D., Kouri, N., and Hirst, W. (2012) Memory's malleability: Its role in shaping collective memory and social identity. *Frontiers in Psychology*, 3. https://doi.org/10.3389/fpsyg.2012.00257.

Bruneau, E. (2016, November–December) Understanding the terrorist mind. *Cerebrum*, 2016. PMID: 28058095

Bruneau, E. (2017) Why we fight. *Psychological Science Agenda*. https://www.apa.org/science/about/psa/2017/12/why-fight

Bruneau, E., Kteily, N., and Laustsen, L. (2018) The unique effects of blatant dehumanization on attitudes and behavior towards Muslim refugees during the European "refugee crisis" across four countries. *European Journal of Social Psychology*, 48(5), 645–662.

Bruneau, E. and Saxe, R. (2010) Attitudes towards the outgroup are predicted by activity in the precuneus in Arabs and Israelis. *NeuroImage*, 52(4), 1704–1711.

Bruneau, E. and Saxe, R. (2012) The power of being heard: The benefits of "perspective-giving" in the context of intergroup conflict. *Journal of Experimental Social Psychology*, 48(4), 855–866.

Buchan, N.R., Grimalda, G., Wilson, R., Brewer, M., Fatas, E., and Foddy, M. (2009) Globalization and human cooperation. *Proceedings of the National Academy of Sciences of the United States of America*, 106(11), 4138–4142.

Bucy, E. (2000) Emotional and evaluative consequences of inappropriate leader displays. *Communication Research*, 27(2), 194–226.

Burnham, T.C. and Johnson, D.D.P. (2005) The biological and evolutionary logic of human cooperation. *Analyse & Kritik*, 27, 113–135.

Burns, J.M. (1978) *Leadership*. New York: Harper & Row.

Butler, E.A., Lee, T.L., and Gross, J.J. (2007) Emotion regulation and culture: Are the social consequences of emotion suppression culture-specific? *Emotion*, 7(1), 30–48.

Butz, S., Kieslich, P.J., and Bless, H. (2017) Why are conservatives happier than liberals? Comparing different explanations based on system justification, multiple group membership, and positive adjustment. *European Journal of Social Psychology*, 47(3), 362–372.

Buvinic, M. and Morrison, A. (1999) *Violence as an obstacle to development*. Washington, DC: Inter-American Development Bank.

Byrne, P. (2017, August 16) Anatomy of terror: What makes normal people become extremists? *New Scientist*.

Cacioppo, J.T. and Decety, J. (2011) Challenges and opportunities in social neuroscience. *Annals of the New York Academy of Sciences*, 1224(1), 162–173.

Cahn, D. (2016, September 21) Former admirals and generals warn Trump is "dangerous" to military and country. *Stars and Stripes*. https://www.stripes.com/news/former-admirals-and-generals-warn-trump-is-dangerous-to-military-and-country-1.430242#.WUe4a8aZNuU

Callimachi, R. (2015, August 13) ISIS enshrines a theology of rape. *New York Times*.

Cannon, W.B. (1915) *Bodily changes in pain, hunger, fear and rage*. New York: D. Appleton.

Carnegie Corporation of New York (1997) Preventing deadly conflict: Final report. https://www.carnegie.org/publications/preventing-deadly-conflict-final-report/

Carr, N. (2015, September 2) How social media is ruining politics. *Politico Magazine*. https://www.politico.com/magazine/story/2015/09/2016-election-social-media-ruining-politics-213104

Chae, D.H., Lincoln, K.D., Adler, N.E., and Syme, S.L. (2010) Do experiences of racial discrimination predict cardiovascular disease among African American men? The moderating role of internalized negative racial group attitudes. *Social Science & Medicine*, 71(6), 1182–1188.

Chang, S.W.C., Gariépy, J.-F., and Platt, M.L. (2013) Neuronal reference frames for social decisions in primate frontal cortex. *Nature Neuroscience*, 16, 243–250.

ChangeFactory (n.d.) Working with cultural differences. https://www.changefactory. com.au/our-thinking/articles/working-with-cultural-differences/

Charney, E. and English, W. (2012) Candidate genes and political behaviour. *American Political Science Review*, 106(1), 1–34.

Chen, C., Burton, M.L., Greenberger, E., and Dmitrieva, J. (1999) Population migration and the variation of dopamine (DRD4) allele frequencies around the globe. *Evolution and Human Behavior*, 20, 309–324.

Cheon, B.K., Livingston, R.W., Hong, Y.Y., and Chiao, J.Y. (2014) Gene × environment interaction on intergroup bias: The role of 5-HTTLPR and perceived outgroup threat. *Social Cognitive and Affective Neuroscience*, 9(9), 1268–1275.

Chi, C. (2019) 51 YouTube stats every video marketer should know in 2019. *HubSpot*. https://blog.hubspot.com/marketing/youtube-stats

Chiao, J.Y. (2009) Cultural neuroscience: A once and future discipline. In J.Y. Chiao (ed.), *Progress in Brain Research* (Vol. 178, pp. 287–304). Amsterdam: Elsevier.

Chiao, J.Y. and Blizinsky, K.D. (2009) Culture–gene coevolution of individualism-collectivism and the serotonin transporter gene. *Proceedings of the Royal Society B: Biological Sciences*, 277(1681). https://doi.org/10.1098/rspb.2009.1650

Chiao, J.Y., Harada, T., Komeda, H., Li, Z., Mano, Y., Saito, D., Parrish, T.B., Sadato, N., and Iidaka, T. (2010) Dynamic cultural influences on neural representations of the Self. *Journal of Cognitive Neuroscience*, 22(1), 1–11.

Chiao, J.Y., Hariri, A.R., Harada, T., Mano, Y., Sadato, N., Parrish, T.B., and Iidaka, T. (2010) Theory and methods in cultural neuroscience. *Social Cognitive and Affective Neuroscience*, 5(2–3), 353–361.

Chiao, J.Y., Iidaka, T., Gordon, H.L., Nogawa, J., Bar, M., Aminoff, E., Sadato, N., and Ambady, N. (2008) Cultural specificity in amygdala response to fear faces. *Journal of Cognitive Neuroscience*, 20, 2167–2174.

Choi, J.K. and Bowles, S. (2007) The coevolution of parochial altruism and war. *Science*, 318(5850), 636–640.

Christakis, N.A. (2008) 2008: What have you changed your mind about? Why? *Edge*. https://www.edge.org/response-detail/10456

Christov-Moore, L. and Iacoboni, M. (2016) Self–other resonance, its control and pro-social inclinations: Brain–behavior relationships. *Human Brain Mapping*, 37(4), 1544–1558.

Church, C., Visser, A., and Johnson, L. (2002) *Single identity work: An approach to conflict resolution in Northern Ireland*. Derry/Londonderry: INCORE.

Ciampaglia, G.L. and Menczer, F. (2018, June 20) Misinformation and biases infect social media, both intentionally and accidentally. *The Conversation*. http://theconversation. com/misinformation-and-biases-infect-social-media-both-intentionally-and-accidentally-97148

Coaching US troops on Iraqi culture. (2007, July 19) *BBC News*. http://news.bbc.co.uk/1/ hi/world/americas/6904842.stm

Cohen, T.R., Montoya, R.M., and Insko, C.A. (2006) Group morality and intergroup relations: Cross-cultural and experimental evidence. *Personal and Social Psychology Bulletin*, 32(11), 1159–1172.

Cole Wright, J. and Baril, G. (2011) The role of cognitive resources in determining our moral intuitions: Are we all liberals at heart? *Journal of Experimental Social Psychology*, 47(5), 1007–1012.

Colgin, L.L., Denninger, T., Fyhn, M., Hafting, T., Bonnevie, T., Jensen, O., Moser, M.B, and Moser, E.I. (2009) Frequency of gamma oscillations routes flow of information in the hippocampus. *Nature*, 462(7271), 353–357.

Consorti, A., Sansevero, G. Torelli, C., Berardi, N., and Sale, A. (2019) From basic visual science to neurodevelopmental disorders: The voyage of environmental enrichment-like stimulation. *Neural Plasticity*, 2019:5653180.

Conway, L.G., III, Suedfeld, P., and Tetlock, P.E. (2001) Integrative complexity and political decisions that lead to war or peace. In D.J. Christie, R.V. Wagner, and D.D. Winter (eds.), *Peace, conflict, and violence: Peace psychology for the 21st century* (pp. 66–75). Englewood Cliffs, NJ: Prentice Hall.

Cook-Greuter, S.R. (1999) Postautonomous ego development: A study of its nature and measurement (habits of mind, transpersonal psychology, worldview). *Dissertation Abstracts International: Section B: The Sciences and Engineering*, 60(6-B), 3000.

Cooper, P. (2019) 28 Twitter stats all marketers need to know in 2020. *Hootsuite*. https://blog.hootsuite.com/twitter-statistics/

Crawshaw, S. (1998, October 11) Even if the bloodbath in Kosovo is averted, Slobodan Milosevic's self-seeking and destabilising quest for power has ensured that everyone will be a loser. *The Independent*. https://www.independent.co.uk/life-style/focus-he-taught-the-serbs-how-to-hate-1177649.html

Creanza, N., Kolodny, O., and Feldman, M.W. (2017) Cultural evolutionary theory: How culture evolves and why it matters. *Proceedings of the National Academy of Sciences of the United States of America*, 114(30), 7782–7789.

Crenshaw, M. (1981) The causes of terrorism. *Comparative Politics*, 13(4), 379–399.

Crick, N.R. and Dodge, K.A. (1996) Social information-processing mechanisms in reactive and proactive aggression. *Child Development*, 67(3), 993–1002.

Critcher, C.R., Huber, M., Ho, A.K., and Koleva, S.P. (2009) Political orientation and ideological inconsistencies: (Dis)comfort with value tradeoffs. *Social Justice Research*, 22, 181–205.

Critcher, C.R., Inbar, Y., and Pizarro, D.A. (2013) How quick decisions illuminate moral character. *Social Psychological and Personality Science*, 4(3), 308–315.

Cross, S., Hardin, E., and Gercek-Swing, B. (2011) The what, how, why, and where of self-construal. *Personality and Social Psychology Review*, 15(2), 142–179.

Cunningham, W.A., Johnson, M.K., Raye, C.L., Gatenby, J.C., Gore, J.C., and Banaji, M.R. (2004) Separable neural components in the processing of black and white faces. *Psychological Science*, 15, 806–813.

Cunningham, W.A. and Zelazo, P.D. (2007) Attitudes and evaluations: A social cognitive neuroscience perspective. *Trends in Cognitive Science*, 11(3), 97–104.

Curley, J. and Ochsner, K. (2017) Neuroscience: Social networks in the brain. *Nature Human Behaviour*, 1(0104). https://www.nature.com/articles/s41562-017-0104

Dacko, S.G. (2008) *The advanced dictionary of marketing*. Oxford: Oxford University Press.

Davies, L. (2011, August 18) England's rioters: Did many '"pillars of the community" take part? *The Guardian*.

Davies, W. (2018) *Nervous states: How feeling took over the world*. London: Jonathan Cape.

Davis, J. (2006) *Women and radical Islamic terrorism: Planners, perpetrators, patrons?* Toronto: Canadian Institute of Strategic Studies.

Davis, J. and Mehta, P.H. (2016) An ideal hormone profile for leadership (Vol. 6). *NeuroLeadership Journal*. https://neuroleadership.com/portfolio-items/an-ideal-hormone-profile-for-leadership-vol-6/

Dawes C.T., Loewen, P.J., Schreiber, D., Simmons, A.N., Flagan, T., McElreath, R., Bokemper, S.E., Fowler, J.H., and Paulus, M.P. (2012) Neural basis of egalitarian behavior. *Proceedings of the National Academy of Sciences of the United States of America*, 109(17), 6479–6483.

Dawkins, R. (1976) *The selfish gene*. Oxford: Oxford University Press.

Dean, K.K. and Koenig, A.M. (2019) Cross-cultural differences and similarities in attribution. In K.D. Keith (ed.), *Cross-cultural psychology: Contemporary themes and perspectives* (2nd ed.). New York: Wiley.

Dearden, L. (2016, October 10). Isis recruiting violent criminals and gang members across Europe in dangerous new "crime-terror nexus." *The Independent*.

Debs, A. and Monteiro, N.P. (2014) Known unknowns: Power shifts, uncertainty, and war. *International Organization*, 68(1), 1–31.

Decety, J., Jackson, P.L., Sommerville, J.A., Chaminade, T., and Meltzoff, A.N. (2004) The neural bases of cooperation and competition: An fMRI investigation. *NeuroImage*, 23(2), 744–751.

Decety, J. and Lamm, C. (2014) The biological bases of empathy. In J.T. Cacioppo and G.G. Berntson (eds.), *Handbook of neuroscience for the behavioral sciences* (p. 23). New York: Wiley.

Decety, J., Pape, R., and Workman, C.I. (2018) A multilevel social neuroscience perspective on radicalization and terrorism. *Social Neuroscience*, 13(5), 511–529.

Decety, J. and Yoder, K.J. (2016) Empathy and motivation for justice: Cognitive empathy and concern, but not emotional empathy, predict sensitivity to injustice for others. *Social Neuroscience*, 11(1), 1–14.

De Dreu, C.K., Greer, L.L., Handgraaf, M.J., Shalvi, S., Van Kleef, G.A., Baas, M., Ten Velden, F.S., Van Dijk, E., and Feith, S.W. (2010). The neuropeptide oxytocin regulates parochial altruism in intergroup conflict among humans. *Science*, 328(5984), 1408–1411. doi: 10.1126/science.1189047. PubMedGov

De Dreu, C.K.W., Greer, L.L., Van Kleef, G.A., Shalvi, S., and Handgraaf, M.J.J. (2011) Oxytocin promotes human ethnocentrism. *Proceedings of the National Academy of Sciences of the United States of America*, 108(4), 1262–1266.

DeLaRosa, B.L., Spence, J.S., Shakal, S.K.M., Motes, M.A., Calley, C.S., Calley, V.I., Hart, J., and Kraut, M.A. (2014) Electrophysiological spatiotemporal dynamics during implicit visual threat processing. *Brain and Cognition*, 91, 54–61.

De Neve, J.E., Mikhaylova, S., Dawes, C.T., Christakis, N.A., and Fowler, J.H. (2013) Born to lead? A twin design and genetic association study of leadership role occupancy. *Leadership Quarterly*, 24(1), 45–60.

Den Hartog, D.N., House, R.J., Hanges, P., Ruiz-Quintanilla, S.A., Dorfman, P.W., Ashkanasy, N.M., et al. (1999) Culture specific and cross culturally generalizable implicit leadership theories. Are attributes of charismatic/transformational leadership universally endorsed? *Leadership Quarterly*, 10(2), 219–256.

Derntl, B., Windischberger, C., Robinson, S., Kryspin-Exner, I., Gur, R.C., Moser, E., and Habel, U. (2009) Amygdala activity to fear and anger in healthy young males is associated with testosterone. *Psychoneuroendocrinology*, 34(5), 687–693.

de Waal, F. (2006) *Primates and philosophers: How morality evolved*. Princeton, NJ: Princeton University Press.

Dfarhud, D., Malmir, M., and Khanahmadi, M. (2014) Happiness & health: The biological factors—systematic review article. *Iranian Journal of Public Health*, 43(11), 1468–1477.

Dickerson, K. (2015 October 30) Here's what happens to your body when something terrifies you. *Business Insider*. https://www.businessinsider.com/what-happens-when-you-are-scared-2015-10

Dickey, C. (2017, April 23) The terrorist tipping point: What pushed the Tsarnaev brothers to violence? *Daily Beast*. https://www.thedailybeast.com/the-terrorist-tipping-point-what-pushed-the-tsarnaev-brothers-to-violence

Dobrin, A. (2017, April 7) We are programmed for fairness. *Psychology Today*. https://www.psychologytoday.com/gb/blog/am-i-right/201704/we-are-programmed-fairness

Dong, Y., Zhang, B., and Tao, Y. (2016) The dynamics of human behavior in the public goods game with institutional incentives. *Scientific Reports*, 6, 28809. https://www.nature.com/articles/srep28809

Doolittle, C. (2016) Liberalism: An evolutionary luxury afforded by decrease in negative stimuli. (Hyperconsumption). https://propertarianism.com/2019/09/27/liberalism-an-evolutionary-luxury-afforded-by-decrease-in-negative-stimuli-hyperconsumption/

Doosje, B., Loseman, A., and van den Bos, K. (2013) Determinants of radicalization of Islamic youth in the Netherlands: Personal uncertainty, perceived injustice, and perceived group threat. *Journal of Social Issues*, 69(3), 586–604.

Doraiswamy, M. (2015) 5 brain technologies that will shape our future. *World Economic Forum*. https://www.weforum.org/agenda/2015/08/5-brain-technologies-future/

Doughty, K. and Ntambara, D.M. (2005) *Resistance and protection: Muslim community actions during the Rwandan cenocide*. Cambridge, MA: CDA Collaborative Learning Projects.

Drury, F. (2015, January 26) Hunted down like animals and sold by their own families for £50,000: Tanzania's albinos hacked apart by witchdoctors who believe their body parts "bring luck" in sick trade "fuelled by the country's elite." *MailOnline*. https://www.dailymail.co.uk/news/article-2922243/Hunted-like-animals-sold-families-75-000-Tanzania-s-albinos-hacked-apart-witchdoctors-believe-body-parts-bring-luck-sick-trade-fuelled-country-s-elite.html

Dugas, M. and Kruglanski, A.W. (2014) The quest for significance model of radicalization: Implications for the management of terrorist detainees. *Behavioral Sciences & the Law*, 32(3), 423–439.

Duke, A.A., Bègue, L., Bell, R., and Eisenlohr-Moul, T. (2013) Revisiting the serotonin-aggression relation in humans: A meta-analysis. *Psychological Bulletin*, 139(5), 1148–1172.

Dumitrescu, D. Gidengil, E., and Stolle, D. (2015) Candidate confidence and electoral appeal: An experimental study of the effect of nonverbal confidence on voter evaluations. *Political Science Research and Methods*, 3(1), 43–52.

Dunbar, R. (2004) Gossip in evolutionary perspective. *Review of General Psychology*, 8(2), 100–110.

Duncan, E.J., Gluckman, P.D., and Dearden, P.K. (2014) Epigenetics, plasticity, and evolution: How do we link epigenetic change to phenotype? *Journal of Experimental Zoology Part B: Molecular and Developmental Evolution*, 322(4), 208–220.

Edkins, B. (2017, August 28) Study: Partisan, ideological politicians attract more Facebook followers. *Forbes*. https://www.forbes.com/sites/brettedkins/2017/08/28/partisan-ideological-politicians-attract-more-facebook-followers-study-finds/#48bab1333fb9

Eggert, J.P. (2018) Female fighters and militants during the Lebanese Civil War: Individual profiles, pathways, and motivations. *Studies in Conflict & Terrorism*. https://doi.org/10.1080/1057610X.2018.1529353

Ehrlich, P.R. (2000) *Human natures: Genes, cultures, and the human prospect.* Washington, DC: Island Press.

Election 2016: Trump voters on why they backed him. (2016, November 9). *BBC News.* https://www.bbc.com/news/election-us-2016-36253275

Elmhirst, S. (2011, October 26) I'd have been ashamed not to join the IRA. *New Statesman.*

England's week of riots. (2011, August 15) *BBC News* https://www.bbc.co.uk/news/uk-14532532

Fan, R., Xu, K., and Zhao, J. (2016) Higher contagion and weaker ties mean anger spreads faster than joy in social media. *Cornell University.* https://arxiv.org/abs/1608.03656

Fazekas, Z. and Littvay, L. (2015) The Importance of context in the genetic transmission of US party identification. *Political Psychology*, 36(4), 361–377.

Fecteau, S., Pascual-Leone, A., Zald, D.H., Liguori, P., Théoret, H., Boggio, P.S., and Fregni, F. (2007) Activation of prefrontal cortex by transcranial direct current stimulation reduces appetite for risk during ambiguous decision making. *Journal of Neuroscience*, 27(23), 6212–6218.

Feddes, A.R., Mann, L., and Doosje, B. (2015) Increasing self-esteem and empathy to prevent violent radicalization: A longitudinal quantitative evaluation of a resilience training focused on adolescents with a dual identity. *Journal of Applied Social Psychology*, 45(7), 400–411.

Federico, C.M., Weber, C.R., Ergun, D., and Hunt, C. (2013) Mapping the connections between politics and morality: The multiple sociopolitical orientations involved in moral intuition. *Political Psychology*, 34(4), 589–610.

Fehr, E. and Fischbacher, U. (2004a) Third-party punishment and social norms. *Evolution and Human Behavior*, 25(2), 63–87.

Fehr, E. and Fischbacher, U. (2004b) Social norms and human cooperation. *Trends in Cognitive Sciences*, 8(4), 185–190.

Fehr, E. and Gächter, S. (2000) Fairness and retaliation: The economics of reciprocity. *Journal of Economic Perspectives*, 14(3), 159–181.

Feinberg, A.P. (2008) Epigenetics at the epicenter of modern medicine. *Journal of the American Medical Association*, 299(11), 1345–1350.

Festinger, L. (1962) Cognitive dissonance. *Scientific American*, 207(4), 93–107.

Fick, M. and Dave, P. (2019) Facebook's flood of languages leave it struggling to monitor content. *Reuters.* https://www.reuters.com/article/us-facebook-languages-insight/facebooks-flood-of-languages-leave-it-struggling-to-monitor-content-idUSKCN1RZ0DW

Figueiredo, A., Martinovic, B., Rees, J., and Licata, L. (2017) Collective memories and present-day intergroup relations: Introduction to the special thematic section. *Journal of Social and Political Psychology*, 5(2), 694–706.

Fincher, C.L., Thornhill, R., Murray, D.R., and Schaller, M. (2008) Pathogen prevalence predicts human cross-cultural variability in individualism/collectivism. *Proceedings of the Royal Society B: Biological Sciences*, 275(1640). https://doi.org/10.1098/rspb.2008.0094

Fischbacher, U., Gächter, S., and Fehr, E. (2001) Are people conditionally cooperative? Evidence from a public goods experiment. *Economics Letters*, 71(3), 397–404.

Fisk, R. (1993, February 8) Bosnia war crimes: "The rapes went on day and night": Robert Fisk, in Mostar, gathers detailed evidence of the systematic sexual assaults on Muslim women by Serbian "White Eagle" gunmen. *The Independent*.

Fitzduff, M. (1989) *From ritual to consciousness—A study of change and progress in Northern Ireland*. PhD thesis, New University of Ulster, Coleraine.

Fitzduff, M. (2010) Women and war in Northern Ireland—a slow growth to power. *South Asian Journal of Peacebuilding*, 3(1). http://wiscomp.org/peaceprints/3-1/3.1.1.pdf

Fitzduff, M. (2013) *Minority women as agents of change in shared societies*. Project Briefing Paper on Women and Shared Societies: Meeting of the Working Group on Double Discrimination, Madrid.

Fitzduff, M. (2016) Lessons learned on trust building in Northern Ireland. In I. Alon and D. Bar-Tal (eds.), *The role of trust in conflict resolution: The Israeli–Palestinian case and beyond* (pp. 41–58). Cham, Switzerland: Springer.

Fitzduff, M. (ed.) (2017) *Why irrational politics appeals: Understanding the allure of Trump*. Santa Barbara, CA: Praeger.

Fitzduff, M. and Stout, C.E. (eds.) (2006) *The psychology of resolving global conflicts: From war to peace*. Westport, CT: Praeger.

Fitzduff, M. and Williams, S. (2019) *Dialogue in divided societies: Skills for working with groups in conflict*. Independently published.

Forsberg, E. and Olsson, L. (2016) Gender inequality and internal conflict. *Oxford Research Encyclopedias*. https://oxfordre.com/politics/view/10.1093/acrefore/9780190228637.001.0001/acrefore-9780190228637-e-34

Foster, R. (2016) "I want my country back": Emotion and Englishness at the Brexit ballotbox. *EU Referendum Analysis*. https://www.referendumanalysis.eu/eu-referendum-zanalysis-2016/section-8-voters/i-want-my-country-back-emotion-and-englishness-at-the-brexit-ballotbox/

Fowler, J. and Schreiber, D. (2008) Biology, politics, and the emerging science of human nature. *Science*, 322(5903), 912–914.

Freeman J.B., Rule, N.O., Adams, R.B. Jr, and Ambady, N. (2009) Culture shapes a mesolimbic response to signals of dominance and subordination that associates with behavior. *NeuroImage*, 47(1), 353–359.

Futures without Violence (2017) What is violent extremism? https://www.futureswithoutviolence.org/wp-content/uploads/FWV_blueprint_3-What-is-VE.pdf

Gambetta, D. and Hertog, S. (2016) *Engineers of jihad: The curious connection between violent extremism and education*. Princeton, NJ: Princeton University Press.

Garagozov, R. (2016) Painful collective memory: Measuring collective memory affect in the Karabakh conflict. *Peace and Conflict*, 22(1), 28–35.

Geher, G. (2015, June 3) Rejecting evolutionary psychology is rejecting evolution: Evolution does not stop at the neck. *Psychology Today*. https://www.psychologytoday.com/us/blog/darwins-subterranean-world/201506/rejecting-evolutionary-psychology-is-rejecting-evolution

Gentry, C. and Sjoberg, L. (2016) Female terrorism and militancy. In J. Richard (ed.), *Handbook of critical terrorism studies* (pp. 145–155). Abingdon, UK: Routledge.

Gerstner, C.R. and Day, D.V. (1994) Cross-cultural comparison of leadership prototypes. *Leadership Quarterly*, 5(2), 121–134.

Giacomin, M. and Jordan, C. (2017) Interdependent and independent self-construal. In V. Zeigler-Hill and T. Shackelford (eds.), *Encyclopedia of personality and individual differences*. Cham, Switzerland: Springer.

Ginges, J., Atran, S., Medin, D., and Shikaki, K. (2007) Sacred bounds on rational resolution of violent political conflict. *Proceedings of the National Academy of Sciences of the United States of America*, 104(18), 7357–7360.

Glover, H. (1985) Guilt and aggression in Vietnam veterans. *American Journal of Social Psychiatry*, 5(1), 15–18.

Goldman, J.G. (2014, April 10) How human culture influences our genetics. *BBC Future*. https://www.bbc.com/future/article/20140410-can-we-drive-our-own-evolution

Golumbia, D. (2018, January 5) Social media has hijacked our brains and threatens global democracy. *Vice*. https://www.vice.com/en_us/article/bjy7ez/social-media-threatens-global-democracy

Goñi, U. (2002) *The real Odessa: Smuggling the Nazis to Perón's Argentina*. London: Granta.

Gordon, I., Martin, C., Feldman, R., and Leckman, J.F. (2011) Oxytocin and social motivation. *Developmental Cognitive Neuroscience*, 1(4), 471–493.

Grabo, A. and van Vugt, M. (2016) Charismatic leadership and the evolution of cooperation. *Evolution and Human Behavior*, 37(5), 399–406.

Grant, A. (2014, January 2) The dark side of emotional intelligence. *The Atlantic*. https://www.theatlantic.com/health/archive/2014/01/the-dark-side-of-emotional-intelligence/282720/

Greene, J. (2011) *Moral tribes: Emotion, reason and the gap between us and them*. London: Penguin.

Grierson, J. (2019, November 3) Isis women driven by more than marriage, research shows. *The Guardian*. https://www.theguardian.com/uk-news/2019/nov/03/isis-women-driven-by-more-than-marriage-research-shows

Grillo, M. (2017) Nationalist politics: The role of predispositions and emotions. In M. Fitzduff (ed.), *Why irrational politics appeals: Understanding the allure of Trump* (pp. 87–106). Santa Barbara, CA: Praeger.

Gross, J.J. (1998) The emerging field of emotion regulation: An integrative review. *Review of General Psychology*, 2(3), 271–299.

Guyon, J. (2018, April 22) In Sri Lanka, Facebook is like the ministry of truth. *Quartz*. https://qz.com/1259010/how-facebook-rumors-led-to-real-life-violence-in-sri-lanka/

Haidt, J. (2006) *The happiness hypothesis: Finding modern truth in ancient wisdom*. New York: Basic Books.

Haidt, J. (2012) *The righteous mind: Why good people are divided by politics and religion*. New York: Pantheon.

Haidt, J. and Joseph, C. (2006) Intuitive ethics: How innately prepared intuitions generate culturally variable virtues. *Daedalus*, 133(4), pp. 55–66.

Hall, E.T. (1976) *Beyond culture*. Garden City, NY: Anchor Press.

Hamilton, D.M. (2015, December 22) Calming your brain during conflict. *Harvard Business Review*. https://hbr.org/2015/12/calming-your-brain-during-conflict

Han, S. and Northoff, G. (2008) Culture-sensitive neural substrates of human cognition: A transcultural neuroimaging approach. *Nature Reviews Neuroscience*, 9, 646–654.

Han, S., Northoff, G., Vogeley, K., Wexler, B.E., Kitayama, S., and Varnum, M.E.W. (2013) A cultural neuroscience approach to the biosocial nature of the human brain. *Annual Review of Psychology*, 64(1), 335–359.

Handley, C. and Mathew, S. (2020) Human large-scale cooperation as a product of competition between cultural groups. *Nature Communications*, 11(702). https://www.nature.com/articles/s41467-020-14416-8

Handley, P. (2018, May 24) US disrupts Russian botnet of 500,000 hacked routers. *PhysOrg*. https://phys.org/news/2018-05-disrupts-russian-botnet-hacked-routers.html

Hänska, M. and Bauchowitz, S. (2017, October) Tweeting for Brexit: How social media influenced the referendum. *LSE Research Online*. http://eprints.lse.ac.uk/84614/1/Hanska-Ahy__tweeting-for-brexit.pdf

Hard-wired: The brain's circuitry for political belief. (2016, December 23) *Science Daily*. www.sciencedaily.com/releases/2016/12/161223115757.htm

Harbath, K. (2018, January 22) Hard questions: Social media and democracy, *Facebook*. https://newsroom.fb.com/news/2018/01/hard-questions-democracy/

Harman, C. (1981) The summer of 1981: A post-riot analysis. *International Socialism*, 2(14), 1–43. www.marxists.org/archive/harman/1981/xx/riots.htm

Harris, S., Sheth, S.A., and Cohen M.S. (2008) Functional neuroimaging of belief, disbelief, and uncertainty. *Annals of Neurology*, 63(2), 141–147.

Hasan, M. (2014, August 21) What the jihadists who bought "Islam for Dummies" on Amazon tell us about radicalisation. *New Statesman*. https://www.newstatesman.com/religion/2014/08/what-jihadists-who-bought-islam-dummies-amazon-tell-us-about-radicalisation

Haslam, N. (2006) Dehumanization: An integrative review. *Personality and Social Psychology Review*, 10(3), 252–264.

Hatemi, P.K. (2013) The influence of major life events on economic attitudes in a world of gene–environment interplay. *American Journal of Political Science*, 57(4), 987–1007.

Hatemi, P.K. and McDermott, R. (2012) The genetics of politics: Discovery, challenges, and progress. *Trends in Genetics*, 28(10), 525–533.

Hatemi, P.K. and McDermott, R. (2016) Give me attitudes. *Annual Review of Political Science*, 19, 331–350.

Hatemi, P.K., McDermott, R., Eaves, L.J., Kendler, K.S., and Neale, M.C. (2013) Fear as a disposition and an emotional state: A genetic and environmental approach to outgroup political preferences. *American Journal of Political Science*, 57(2), 279–293.

Hatemi, P.K., Medland, S.E., Klemmensen R., Oskarsson, S., Littvay, L., Dawes, C.T., Verhulst, B., McDermott, R., Nørgaard, A.S., Klofstad, C.A., Christensen, K., Johannesson, M., Magnusson, P.K., Eaves, L.J., and Martin, N.G. (2014) Genetic influences on political ideologies: Twin analyses of 19 measures of political ideologies from five democracies and genome-wide findings from three populations. *Behavior Genetics*, 44(3), 282–294.

Haynes, T. (2018) Dopamine, smartphones & you: A battle for your time. *Science in the News, Harvard Graduate School of the Arts and Sciences*. http://sitn.hms.harvard.edu/flash/2018/dopamine-smartphones-battle-time/

He, Q., Turel, O., and Bechara, A. (2017) Brain anatomy alterations associated with social networking site (SNS) addiction. *Nature Scientific Reports*, 7(45064). https://www.nature.com/articles/srep45064

Hedden, T., Ketay, S., Aron, A., Markus, H.R., and Gabrieli, J.D. (2008) Cultural influences on neural substrates of attentional control. *Psychological Science*, 19(1), 12–17.

Hedges, C. (2002) *War is a force that gives us meaning*. New York: PublicAffairs.

Henrich, J. and McElreath, R. (2012) Dual-inheritance theory: The evolution of human cultural capacities and cultural evolution. In L. Barrett and R. Dunbar (eds.), *Oxford handbook of evolutionary psychology*. New York: Oxford University Press.

Herzmann, G., Willenbockel, V., Tanaka, J.W., and Curran, T. (2011) The neural correlates of memory encoding and recognition for own-race and other-race faces. *Neuropsychologia*, 49(11), 3103–3115.

Heuveline, P. (2001) The demographic analysis of mortality crises: The case of Cambodia, 1970–1979. In National Research Council, *Forced migration and mortality* (pp. 102–105). Washington, DC: National Academies Press.

Hibbing, J., Smith, K., and Alford, J. (2014) *Predisposed: Liberals, conservatives, and the biology of political differences*. New York: Routledge.

Hitler comes to power. (n.d.) *Holocaust encyclopedia* https://encyclopedia.ushmm.org/content/en/article/hitler-comes-to-power

Hoffer, E. (1951) *The true believer: Thoughts on the nature of mass movements*. New York: Harper & Brothers.

Hoffman, B. (2001, December) Gaza City: All you need is love. How the terrorists stopped terrorism. *Atlantic Monthly*. https://www.theatlantic.com/past/docs/issues/2001/12/hoffman.htm

Hofstede, G. (1997) *Cultures and organizations: Software of the mind*. London: McGraw-Hill.

Hofstede, G. (2001) *Culture's consequences: Comparing values, behaviors, institutions, and organizations across nations* (2nd ed.). Thousand Oaks, CA: SAGE.

Hofstede, G. (2011) Dimensionalizing cultures: The Hofstede model in context. *Online Readings in Psychology and Culture*, 2(1). https://doi.org/10.9707/2307-0919.1014

Hofstede, G. and Fink, G. (2007) Culture: Organisations, personalities and nations: Gerhard Fink interviews Geert Hofstede. *European Journal of International Management*, 1(1–2).

Hofstede, G., Hofstede, G.J., and Minkov, M. (2010) *Cultures and organizations: Software of the mind* (3rd ed.). New York: McGraw-Hill.

Hofstede Insights (n.d.) Country comparison. https://www.hofstede-insights.com/country-comparison/

Hogan, R. (2006) *Personality and the fate of organizations*. Hillsdale, NJ: Erlbaum.

Holbrook, C., Izuma, K., Deblieck, C., Fessler, D.M.T., and Iacoboni, M. (2015) Neuromodulation of group prejudice and religious belief. *Social Cognitive and Affective Neuroscience*, 11(3), 387–394.

Holman, E.A., Garfin, D.R., and Cohen Silver, R. (2019) Media's role in broadcasting acute stress following the Boston Marathon bombings. *Proceedings of the National Academy of Sciences of the United States of America*, 111(1), 93–98.

Holmes, A. (2018) G2B reviews: Epigenetics, epitranscriptomics, microRNAs and more: Emerging approaches to the study of genes, brain and behavior. *Genes, Brain, and Behavior*, 17(3), e12453.

Holt, S., and Machnyikova, Z. (2013) Culture for shared societies. In M. Fitzduff (ed.), *Public policies in shared societies*. Basingstoke, UK: Palgrave Macmillan.

Horgan, J. (2014) *The psychology of terrorism* (2nd ed.). New York: Routledge.

Horowitz, M.C., Stam, A.C., and Ellis, C.M. (2016) *Why leaders fight*. New York: Cambridge University Press.

House, B.R., Silk, J.B., Henrich, J., Barrett, H.C., Scelza, B.A., Boyette, A.H., Hewlett, B.S., McElreath, R., and Laurence, S. (2013) Ontogeny of prosocial behavior across diverse societies. *Proceedings of the National Academy of Sciences of the United States of America*, 110(36), 14586–14591.

How culture colors the way the mind works. (2000, August 1) *Michigan News*. https://news.umich.edu/how-culture-colors-the-way-the-mind-works/

Hudson, R.A. (1999) *The sociology and psychology of terrorism: Who becomes a terrorist and why*. Washington, DC: Library of Congress.

Huemer, M. (n.d.) Why people are irrational about politics. *Internet Archive*. https://web.archive.org/web/20170516125446/

Human Rights Watch. (2004, November 11) Sri Lanka: Tamil Tigers forcibly recruit child soldiers. https://www.hrw.org/news/2004/11/11/sri-lanka-tamil-tigers-forcibly-recruit-child-soldiers#

Hur, Y.-M. and Rushton, J.P. (2007) Genetic and environmental contributions to prosocial behaviour in 2- to 9-year-old South Korean twins. *Biology Letters*, 3(6). https://doi.org/10.1098/rsbl.2007.0365

Hutchinson, M. (2020, January 30) Facebook climbs to 2.5 billion monthly active users, but rising costs impede income growth. *Social Media Today*. https://www.socialmediatoday.com/news/facebook-climbs-to-25-billion-monthly-active-users-but-rising-costs-imped/571358/

Iacobini, M. (2009) Imitation, empathy, and mirror neurons. *Annual Review of Psychology*, 60, 653–670.

IDA Ireland (2020) Doing business here: Medical technology. https://www.idaireland.com/doing-business-here/industry-sectors/medical-technology

Inclusive Security (n.d.) Why women? https://www.inclusivesecurity.org/why-women/

Ingram, D. (2018, March 20) Factbox: Who is Cambridge Analytica and what did it do? *Reuters*. https://www.reuters.com/article/us-facebook-cambridge-analytica-factbox/factbox-who-is-cambridge-analytica-and-what-did-it-do-idUSKBN1GW07F

Institute for Economics and Peace (2019) *Global Terrorism Index 2019: Measuring the impact of terrorism*. Sydney, Australia: Institute for Economics and Peace.

Irwin, C. (2006) The Northern Ireland "peace polls." *Irish Political Studies*, 21(1), 1–14.

ISAF Public Affairs Office (2010) Gen. Petraeus updates guidance on use of force. *U.S. Central Command*. https://www.centcom.mil/MEDIA/NEWS-ARTICLES/News-Article-View/Article/884119/gen-petraeus-updates-guidance-on-use-of-force/

Ito, T.A. and Urland, G.R. (2005) The influence of processing objectives on the perception of faces: An ERP study of race and gender perception. *Cognitive, Affective, & Behavioral Neuroscience*, 5(1), 21–36.

Jacobson, M. (2010) Terrorist financing and the internet. *Studies in Conflict and Terrorism*, 33(4), 353–363.

Jaeggi, A.V., Trumble, B.C., Kaplan, H.S., and Gurven, M. (2015) Salivary oxytocin increases concurrently with testosterone and time away from home among returning Tsimane' hunters. *Biology Letters*, 11(3). https://doi.org/10.1098/rsbl.2015.0058

Jost, J.T. (2017, June) A theory of system justification: Is there a nonconscious tendency to defend, bolster and justify aspects of the societal status quo? *American Psychological Association Science Brief* https://www.apa.org/science/about/psa/2017/06/system-justification

Jost, J.T. and Amodio, D.M. (2012) Political ideology as motivated social cognition: Behavioral and neuroscientific evidence. *Motivation and Emotion*, 36(1), 55–64.

Jost, J.T., Gaucher, D., and Stern, C. (2015) "The world isn't fair": A system justification perspective on social stratification and inequality. In M. Mikulincer, P.R. Shaver, J.F.

Dovidio, and J.A. Simpson (eds.), *APA handbook of personality and social psychology* (Vol. 2, pp. 317–340). Washington, DC: American Psychological Association.

Jost, J.T., Langer, M., Badaan, V., Azevedo, F., Etchezahar, E., Ungaretti, J., and Hennes, E.P. (2017) Ideology and the limits of self-interest: System justification motivation and conservative advantages in mass politics. *Translational Issues in Psychological Science*, 3(3), e1–e26.

Jost, J.T., Ledgerwood, A., and Hardin, C.D. (2008a) Shared reality, system justification, and the relational basis of ideological beliefs. *Social and Personality Psychology Compass*, 2, 171–186.

Jost, J., Nam, H.H., Amodio, D., and Van Bavel, J. (2014) Political neuroscience: The beginning of a beautiful friendship. *Political Psychology*, 35, S1, 3–42.

Jost, J.T., Nosek, B.A., and Gosling, S.D. (2008b) Ideology: Its resurgence in social, personality, and political psychology, *Perspectives on Psychological Science*, 3(2), 126–136.

Judge, T. and Piccolo, R. (2004) Transformational and transactional leadership: A meta-analytic test of their relative validity. *Journal of Applied Psychology*, 89(5), 755–768.

Jung, N., Wranke, C., Hamburger, K., and Knauff, M. (2014) How emotions affect logical reasoning: Evidence from experiments with mood-manipulated participants, spider phobics, and people with exam anxiety. *Frontiers in Psychology*. https://doi.org/10.3389/fpsyg.2014.00570

Kachel, S., Steffens, M.C., and Niedlich, C. (2016) Traditional masculinity and femininity: Validation of a new scale assessing gender roles. *Frontiers in Psychology*. https://doi.org/10.3389/fpsyg.2016.00956/full

Kahneman, D. (2011) *Thinking, fast and slow*. New York: Farrar, Straus and Giroux.

Kahneman, D., Knetsch, J.L., and Thaler, R.H. (1986) Fairness and the assumptions of economics. *Journal of Business*, 59(4), S285–S300.

Kakkar, H. and Sivanathan, N. (2017) When the appeal of a dominant leader is greater than a prestige leader. *Proceedings of the National Academy of Sciences of the United States of America*, 114(26), 6734–6739.

Kaldor, M. (2012) *New and old wars: Organized violence in a global era*. Cambridge, UK: Polity Press.

Kanai, R., Feilden, T., Firth, C., and Rees, G. (2011) Political orientations are correlated with brain structure in young adults. *Current Biology*, 21(8), 677–680.

Kaplan, J.T., Gimbel, S.I., and Harris, S. (2016) Neural correlates of maintaining one's political beliefs in the face of counterevidence. *Scientific Reports*, 6(39589). https://www.nature.com/articles/srep39589

Kaska, K., Osula, A.-M., and Stinissen, J. (2013) The Cyber Defence Unit of the Estonian Defence League: Legal, policy and organisational analysis. *NATO Cooperative Cyber Defence Centre of Excellence*. https://ccdcoe.org/uploads/2018/10/CDU_Analysis.pdf

Kassam, K.S., Markey, A.R., Cherkassky, V.L., Loewenstein, G., and Just, M.A. (2013) Identifying emotions on the basis of neural activation. *PLoS One*, 8(6), e66032.

Kellow, C.L. and Steeves, H.L. (1998) The role of radio in the Rwandan genocide. *Journal of Communication*, 48(3), 107–128.

Kemp, A.H. and Guastella, A.J. (2011) The role of oxytocin in human affect: A novel hypothesis. *Current Directions in Psychological Science*, 20(4), 222–231.

Kim, H.S., Sherman, D.K., Sasaki, J.Y., Xu, J., Chu, T.Q., Ryu, C., Suh, E.M., Graham, K., and Taylor, S.E. (2010) Culture, distress, and oxytocin receptor polymorphism (OXTR) interact to influence emotional support seeking. *Proceedings of the National Academy of Sciences of the United States of America*, 107(36), 15717–15721.

King, B.J. (2014) Feeling down? Watching this will help. *NPR: 13.7 Cosmos & Culture.* https://www.npr.org/sections/13.7/2014/02/27/283348422/that-s-unfair-you-say-this-monkey-can-relate?t=1578576937920&t=1584459790973

Kirsch, P., Esslinger, C., Chen, Q., Mier, D., Lis, S., Siddhanti, S., Gruppe, H., Mattay, V.S., Gallhofer, B., and Meyer-Lindenberg, A. (2005) Oxytocin modulates neural circuitry for social cognition and fear in humans. *Journal of Neuroscience*, 25(49), 11489–11493.

Klavina, L. and van Zomeren, M. (2018) Protesting to protect 'us' and/or 'them'? Explaining why members of third groups are willing to engage in collective action. *Group Processes & Intergroup Relations*, 23(1), 140–160.

Klein, R.A. (2011) *Sociality as the human condition: Anthropology in economic, philosophical and theological perspective.* Leiden, The Netherlands: Brill.

Klemmensen, R., Hatemi, P.K., Hobolt, S.B., Skytthe, A., and Nørgaard Asbjørn, S. (2012) Heritability in political interest and efficacy across cultures: Denmark and the United States. *Twin Research and Human Genetics*, 15(1), 15–20.

Klofstad, C.A., Anderson, R.C., and Nowicki, S. (2015) Perceptions of competence, strength, and age influence voters to select leaders with lower-pitched voices. *PLoS One*, 10(8), e0133779.

Knafo-Noam, A., Uzefovsky, F., Israel, S., Davidov, M., Zahn-Waxler, C. (2015) The pro-social personality and its facets: Genetic and environmental architecture of mother-reported behavior of 7-year-old twins. *Frontiers in Psychology*, 6(112). https://doi.org/10.3389/fpsyg.2015.00112

Kobayashi, C., Glover, G.H., and Temple, E. (2006) Cultural and linguistic influence on neural bases of "theory of mind": An fMRI study with Japanese bilinguals. *Brain and Language*, 98(2), 210–220.

Kohlberg, L., Levine, C., and Hewer, A. (1983) *Moral stages: A current formulation and a response to critics.* New York: Karger.

Koppensteiner, M., and Grammer, K. (2010) Motion patterns in political speech and their influence on personality ratings. *Journal of Research in Personality*, 44(3), 374–379.

Korostelina, K.V. (2014) Insulter Trump: A bonus for his followers? In M. Fitzduff and C.E. Stout (eds.), *Psychological approaches to dealing with conflict and war* (pp. 153–171). Westport, CT: Greenwood Press.

Kosfeld, M., Heinrichs, M., Zak, P.J., Fischbacher, U., and Fehr, E. (2005) Oxytocin increases trust in humans. *Nature*, 435, 673–676.

Koski, J.E., Xie, H., and Olson, I.R. (2015) Understanding social hierarchies: The neural and psychological foundations of status perception. *Social Neuroscience*, 10(5), 527–550.

Kossowska, M., Szwed, P., Wronka, E., Czarnek, G., and Wyczesany, M. (2016) Anxiolytic function of fundamentalist beliefs: Neurocognitive evidence. *Personality and Individual Differences*, 101, 390–395.

Krill, A. and Platek, S.M. (2009) In-group and out-group membership mediates anterior cingulate activation to social exclusion. *Frontiers in Evolutionary Neuroscience*, 1(1). https://doi.org/10.3389/neuro.18.001.2009

Kruglanski, A.W. (2014, October 28) Psychology not theology: Overcoming ISIS' secret appeal. *E-International Relations.* https://www.e-ir.info/2014/10/28/psychology-not-theology-overcoming-isis-secret-appeal/

Kruglanski, A.W. and Webster, D.M. (1996) Motivated closing of the mind: "Seizing" and "freezing." *Psychological Review*, 103(2), 263–283.

Kteily, N., Bruneau, E., Waytz, A., and Cotterill, S. (2015) The ascent of man: Theoretical and empirical evidence for blatant dehumanization. *Journal of Personality and Social Psychology*, 109(5), 901–931.

Kteily, N., Hodson, G., and Bruneau, E. (2016) They see us as less than human: Metadehumanization predicts intergroup conflict via reciprocal dehumanization. *Journal of Personality and Social Psychology*, 110(3), 343–370.

Kubota, J.T., Banaji, M.R., and Phelps, E.A. (2012) The neuroscience of race. *Nature Neuroscience*, 15, 940–948.

Kysar, D.A. and Salzman, J. (2005) *Environmental tribalism*. Legal Studies Research Paper Series. Ithaca, NY: Cornell Law School.

Lack, J. and Bogacz, F. (2012) The neurophysiology of ADR and process design: A new approach to conflict prevention and resolution? In A.W. Rovine (ed.), *Contemporary issues in international arbitration and mediation: The Fordham Papers* (pp. 341–382). Leiden, The Netherlands: Brill Nijhoff.

Lakens, D. (2016) Grounding social embodiment. *Social Cognition*. In D.C. Molden (ed.), *Understanding priming effects in social psychology* (pp. 175–190). New York: Guilford Press.

Laland, K.N., Odling-Smee, J., and Myles, S. (2010) How culture shaped the human genome: Bringing genetics and the human sciences together. *Nature Reviews Genetics*, 11(2), 137–148.

Lamm, C., Decety, J., and Singer, T. (2011) Meta-analytic evidence for common and distinct neural networks associated with directly experienced pain and empathy for pain. *NeuroImage*, 54, 2492–2502.

Laustsen, L. and Petersen, M.B. (2015) Does a competent leader make a good friend? Conflict, ideology and the psychologies of friendship and followership. *Evolution and Human Behavior*, 36(4), 286–293.

Lazarus, S. (2019, January 27) Women. Life. Freedom: Female fighters of Kurdistan. *CNN*. https://edition.cnn.com/2019/01/27/homepage2/kurdish-female-fighters/index.html

Lessig, L. (1995) The regulation of social meaning. *University of Chicago Law Review*, 62(3), 1.

Lewis, G.J., Kanai, R., Bates, T.C., and Rees, G. (2012) Moral values are associated with individual differences in regional brain volume. *Journal of Cognitive Neuroscience*, 24(8), 1657–1663.

Licata, L. and Klein, O. (2005) Regards croisés sur un passé commun: Anciens colonisés et anciens coloniaux face à l'action belge au Congo [Crossed glances at a common past: Former colonized and colonizer perspectives regarding the Belgian action in the Congo]. In M. Sanchez-Mazas and L. Licata (eds.), *L'Autre: Regards psychosociaux* [*The other: Psychosocial perspectives*] (pp. 241–278). Grenoble: Presses Universitaires de Grenoble.

Lin, L.C. and Telzer, E.H. (2018) An introduction to cultural neuroscience. In J.M. Causadias, E.H. Telzer, and N.A. Gonzales (eds.), *The handbook of culture and biology* (pp. 943–1045). New York: Wiley.

Lindner, E.G. (2006) Humiliation, killing, war, and gender. In M. Fitzduff and C.E. Stout (eds.), *The psychology of resolving global conflicts: From war to peace*. Westport, CT: Praeger.

Lipman-Blumen, J. (2006) *The allure of toxic leaders: Why we follow destructive bosses and corrupt politicians—and how we can survive them*. Oxford: Oxford University Press.

Little, A.C., Roberts, S.C., Jones, B.C., and DeBruine, L.M. (2012) The perception of attractiveness and trustworthiness in male faces affects hypothetical voting decisions differently in wartime and peacetime scenarios. *Quarterly Journal of Experimental Psychology*, 65(10), 2018–2032.

Liu, X., Liu, S., Huang, R., Chen, X., Xie, Y., Ma, R., Luo, Y., Bu, J., and Zhang, X. (2018) Neuroimaging studies reveal the subtle difference among social network size measurements and shed light on new directions. *Frontiers in Neuroscience*, 12(461). https://doi.org/10.3389/fnins.2018.00461/full

Liu, Y., Lin, W., Xu, P., Zhang, D., and Luo, Y. (2015) Neural basis of disgust perception in racial prejudice. *Human Brain Mapping*, 36(12), 5275–5286.

Livingston, R.W. and Drwecki B.B. (2007) Why are some individuals not racially biased? Susceptibility to affective conditioning predicts nonprejudice toward blacks. *Psychological Science*, 18(9), 816–823.

Livingstone Smith, David (2007) *Why we lie: The evolutionary roots of deception and the unconscious mind*. New York: St Martin's Press.

Lock, A. (2011, August 9) Insurers say London riot losses "well over £100m." *City A.M.*

Lord, R.G. and Brown, D.J. (2003) *Leadership processes and follower self-identity*. New York: Psychology Press.

Lord, R.G. Foti, R.J., and De Vader, C.L. (1984) A test of leadership categorization theory: Internal structure, information processing, and leadership perceptions. *Organizational Behavior and Human Performance*, 34(3), 343–378.

Lord, R.G. and Maher K.J. (1991) *Leadership and information processing: Linking perceptions and performance*. Boston: Unwin Hyman.

Ludeke, S., Johnson, W., and Bouchard, T.J. Jr (2013) "Obedience to traditional authority": A heritable factor underlying authoritarianism, conservatism and religiousness. *Personality and Individual Differences*, 55(4), 375–380.

Lunz, K. and Dier, A. (2019) CFFP co-founder Kristina Lunz speaks with Aleksandra Dier, the gender expert at the United Nations Counter-Terrorism Committee Executive Directorate. *Center for Feminist Foreign Policy*. https://centreforfeministforeignpolicy. org/interviews/2019/12/21/aleksandra-dier

Luthans, F., Peterson, S.J., and Ibrayeva, E. (1998) The potential for the "dark side" of leadership in post-communist countries. *Journal of World Business*, 33, 185–201.

Ma, Q., Pei, G., and Jin, J. (2015) What makes you generous? The influence of rural and urban rearing on social discounting in China. *PloS One*, 10(7), e0133078.

Maccoby, M. (2004, September) Why people follow the leader: The power of transference. *Harvard Business Review*. https://hbr.org/2004/09/why-people-follow-the-leader-the-power-of-transference%20Michael%20Maccoby

Mach, P. (2016) Social media used to fuel South Sudan's civil war. *Anadolu Agency*. https:// www.aa.com.tr/en/africa/social-media-used-to-fuel-south-sudans-civil-war-/655493

MacNair, R.M. (2006) Violence begets violence: The consequences of violence become causation. In M. Fitzduff and C.E. Stout (eds.), *The psychology of resolving global conflicts: From war to peace*. Westport, CT: Praeger.

Makhanova, A., Miller, S.L., and Maner, J.K. (2015) Germs and the out-group: Chronic and situational disease concerns affect intergroup categorization. *Evolutionary Behavioral Sciences*, 9(1), 8–19.

Malefakis, M.A. (2019) Social media dynamics in Boko Haram's terrorist insurgence. *Toda Peace Institute*. https://toda.org/assets/files/resources/policy-briefs/t-pb-50_medinat-a.-malefakis_social-media-dynamics-and-boko-harams-terrorist-insurgence.pdf

Mameli, M. (2004) Nongenetic selection and nongenetic inheritance. *British Journal for the Philosophy of Science*, 55(1), 35–71.

Mann, T.C. and Ferguson, M.J. (2015) Can we undo our first impressions? The role of reinterpretation in reversing implicit evaluations. *Journal of Personality and Social Psychology*, 108(6), 823–849.

Margolin, D. (2016) A Palestinian woman's place in terrorism: Organized perpetrators or individual actors? *Studies in Conflict & Terrorism*, 39(10), 912–934.

Markus, H.R. and Kitayama, S. (1991) Culture and the self: Implications for cognition, emotion, and motivation. *Psychological Review*, 98(2), 224–253.

Marsh, J., Mendoza-Denton, R., and Smith, J.A. (2010) *Are we born racist? New insights from neuroscience and positive psychology*. Boston: Beacon Press.

Marsh, N., Scheele, D., Feinstein, J.S., Gerhardt, H., Strang, S., Maier, W., and Hurlemann, R. (2017) Oxytocin-enforced norm compliance reduces xenophobic outgroup rejection. *Proceedings of the National Academy of Sciences of the United States of America*, 114(35), 9314–9319.

Mason, M.F. and Morris, M.W. (2010) Culture, attribution and automaticity: A social cognitive neuroscience view. *Social Cognitive and Affective Neuroscience*, 5(2–3), 292–306.

Mateos-Aparicio, P. and Rodriguez-Moreno, A. (2019) The impact of studying brain plasticity. *Frontiers in Cellular Neuroscience*, 13(66). https://doi.org/10.3389/fncel.2019.00066

Mattan, B.D., Wei, K.Y., Cloutier, J., and Kubota, J.T (2018) The social neuroscience of race-based and status-based prejudice. *Current Opinion in Psychology*, 24, 27–34.

McAdams, D.P. (2013) The psychological self as actor, agent, and author. *Perspectives on Psychological Science*, 8(3), 272–295.

McAllister, B. and Schmid, A.P. (2011) Theories of terrorism. In A.P. Schmid (ed.), *The Routledge handbook of terrorism research*. New York: Routledge.

McCann, S.J. (1992) Alternative formulas to predict the greatness of U.S. presidents: Personological, situational, and zeitgeist factors. *Journal of Personality and Social Psychology*, 62(3), 469–479.

McClelland, D.C. (1975) *Power: The inner experience*. New York: Irvington.

McCloskey, J. (2015) *A fearless life*. Self-published.

McDermott, J. (2012, June 17) Gold overtakes drugs as source of Colombia rebel funds. *BBC News*. https://www.bbc.com/news/world-latin-america-18396920

McFadyen, S. and Pallenberg, M. (2016, April 13) "Blonde, blue-eyed girls are particularly popular," says ISIS sex slave captured in Iraq. *Daily Express*. https://www.express.co.uk/news/world/699543/Chilling-warning-as-ISIS-hunt-blonde-blue-eyed-girls-to-become-sex-slaves

McMahan, D.L. (2009) *The making of Buddhist modernism*. Oxford: Oxford University Press.

Mendez, M.F. (2011) A neurology of the conservative–liberal dimension of political ideology. *Journal of Neuropsychiatry and Clinical Neurosciences*, 29(2), 86–94.

Mercier, H. and Sperber, D. (2012) "Two heads are better" stands to reason. *Science*, 336(6084), 979.

Mercy Corps (2016) Motivations and empty promises: Voices of former Boko Haram combatants and Nigerian youth 2016. https://www.mercycorps.org/research-resources/boko-haram-nigerian

Mercy Corps (2019) The weaponization of social media. https://www.mercycorps.org/research-resources/weaponization-social-media

Meshi, D., Tamir, D.I., and Heekeren, H. (2015) The emerging neuroscience of social media. *Trends in Cognitive Sciences*, 19(12), 771–782.

Mesquita, B. and Leu, J. (2007) The cultural psychology of emotion. In S. Kitayama and D. Cohen (eds.), *Handbook of cultural psychology* (pp. 734–759). New York: Guilford Press.

Mickiewicz, T. and Rebmann, A. (2020) Entrepreneurship as trust. *Foundations and Trends in Entrepreneurship*, 16(3), 244–309.

The middle class "rioters" revealed: The millionaire's daughter, the aspiring musician and the organic chef all in the dock. (2011, September 2) *Daily Mail.* https://www.dailymail.co.uk/news/article-2025068/UK-riots-Middle-class-rioters-revealed-including-Laura-Johnson-Natasha-Reid-Stefan-Hoyle.html

Mihailidis, P. and Viotty, S. (2017) Spreadable spectacle in digital culture: Civic expression, fake news, and the role of media literacies in "post-fact" society. *American Behavioral Scientist*, 61(4), 441–454.

Miles, T. (2018, March 12) U.N. investigators cite Facebook role in Myanmar crisis. *Reuters.* https://uk.reuters.com/article/us-myanmar-rohingya-facebook/u-n-investigators-cite-facebook-role-in-myanmar-crisis-idUKKCN1GO2PN

Milgram, S. (1963) Behavioral study of obedience. *Journal of Abnormal and Social Psychology*, 67, 371–378.

Millar, M.C. (2012) Magnetic stimulation: A new approach to treating depression? *Harvard Medical School.* https://www.health.harvard.edu/blog/magnetic-stimulation-a-new-approach-to-treating-depression-201207265064

Mischel, W. (1973) Toward a cognitive social learning reconceptualization of personality. *Psychological Review*, 80(4), 252–283.

Mitchell, A., Brown, H., and Guskin, E. (2012, November 28) The role of social media in the Arab uprisings. *Pew Research Center.* https://www.journalism.org/2012/11/28/role-social-media-arab-uprisings/

Mobbs, D., Hagan, C.C., Dalgleish, T., Silston, B., and Prévost, C. (2015) The ecology of human fear: Survival optimization and the nervous system. *Frontiers in Neuroscience*, 9(55). https://doi.org/10.3389/fnins.2015.00055/full

Molina-Morales, F.X. and Martinez-Fernandez, M.T. (2009) Too much love in the neighborhood can hurt: How an excess of intensity and trust in relationships may produce negative effects on firms. *Strategic Management Journal*, 30(9), 1013–1023.

Mooney, C. (2012a, May 1) Inside the political brain. *The Atlantic.* https://www.theatlantic.com/politics/archive/2012/05/inside-the-political-brain/256483/

Mooney, C. (2012b) *The Republican brain: The science of why they deny science—and reality.* New York: Wiley.

Morrison, S., Decety, J., and Molenberghs, P. (2012) The neuroscience of group membership. *Neuropsychologia*, 50(8), 2114–2120.

Murray, G.R. (2017) Mass political behaviour and biology. In S.A. Peterson and A. Somit (eds.), *Handbook of biology and politics* (pp. 1013–1023). Cheltenham, UK: Edward Elgar.

Nam, H.H., Jost, J.T., Kaggen, L., Campbell-Meiklejohn, D., and Van Bavel, J.J. (2018) Amygdala structure and the tendency to regard the social system as legitimate and desirable. *Nature Human Behaviour*, 2, 133–138.

Navarrete, C.D. and Fessler, D.M.T. (2006) Disease avoidance and ethnocentrism: The effects of disease vulnerability and disgust sensitivity on intergroup attitudes. *Evolution and Human Behavior*, 27(4), 270–282.

Nehme, M. (2016) Fundamentalism, terrorism and political instability: Socio-psychological approach. *Lebanese Army*. https://www.lebarmy.gov.lb/en/content/fundamentalism-terrorism-and-political-instability-socio-psychological-approach

Netting, R.M. (1993) *Smallholders, householders: Farm families and the ecology of intensive, sustainable agriculture*. Stanford, CA: Stanford University Press.

Ng, S.H., Han, S., Mao, L., and Lai, J.C.L. (2010) Dynamic bicultural brains: fMRI study of their flexible neural representation of self and significant others in response to culture primes. *Asian Journal of Social Psychology*, 13(2), 83–91.

Nicas, J. (2018, February 7) How YouTube drives people to the internet's darkest corners. *Wall Street Journal*.

Nisbett, R.E. (2003) *The geography of thought: How Asians and Westerners think differently . . . and why*. New York: Free Press.

Nisbett, R.E., Peng, K., Choi, I., and Norenzayan, A. (2001) Culture and systems of thought: Holistic versus analytic cognition. *Psychological Review*, 108(2), 291–310.

Nowak, M.A., Tarnita, C.E., and Wilson, E.O. (2010) The evolution of eusociality. *Nature*, 466(7310), 1057–1062.

Nowrojee, B. (1996) *Shattered lives: Sexual violence during the Rwandan genocide and its aftermath*. New York: Human Rights Watch.

N-Peace Network (2019) *Next generation women, peace and security: N-Peace 2018–2019 edition*. New York: UNDP.

O'Gorman, R., Henrich, J., and Van Vugt, M. (2008) Constraining free riding in public goods games: Designated solitary punishers can sustain human cooperation. *Proceedings of the Royal Society B: Biological Sciences*, 276(1655). https://doi.org/10.1098/rspb.2008.1082

Olson, J.M. and Jang, K.L. (2001) The heritability of attitudes: A study of twins. *Journal of Personality and Social Psychology*, 80(6), 845–860.

Ong, J.C. and Cabañes, J.V.A. (2018) Architects of networked disinformation: Behind the scenes of troll accounts and fake news production in the Philippines. *Scholarworks@ UMassAmherst*. https://scholarworks.umass.edu/communication_faculty_pubs/74/

Optimizing for engagement: Understanding the use of persuasive technology on Internet platforms: *Written testimony to United States Senate Committee on Commerce, Science, and Transportation Subcommittee on Communications, Technology, Innovation and the Internet*. 116th Congr. (2019) (Testimony of T. Harris). https://www.commerce.senate.gov/services/files/96E3A739-DC8D-45F1-87D7-EC70A368371D

Orey, B.D.A. and Park, H. (2012) Nature, nurture, and ethnocentrism in the Minnesota Twin Study. *Twin Research and Human Genetics*, 15(1), 71–73.

Oxley, D.R., Smith, K.B., Alford, J.R., Hibbing, M.V., Miller, J.L., Scalora, M.J., Hatemi, P.K., and Hibbing, J.R. (2008) Political attitudes vary with physiological traits. *Science*, 321(5896), 1667–1670.

Padilla, A., Hogan, R., and Kaiser, R.B. (2007) The toxic triangle: Destructive leaders, susceptible followers, and conducive environments. *Leadership Quarterly*, 18(3), 176–194.

Paluck, E. and Green, D.P. (2009) Prejudice reduction: What works? A review and assessment of research and practice. *Annual Review of Psychology*, 60, 339–367.

Panno, A., Carrus, G., Brizi, A., Maricchiolo, F., Giacomantonio, M., and Mannetti, L. (2018) Need for cognitive closure and political ideology: Predicting pro-environmental preferences and behavior. *Social Psychology*, 49(2), 103–112.

Park, D.C. and Huang, C.-M. (2010) Culture wires the brain: A cognitive neuroscience perspective. *Perspectives on Psychological Science*, 5(4), 391–400.

Paton Walsh, N., Abdelaziz, S., Phillips, M., and Hasan, M. (2017, July 17). ISIS brides flee caliphate as noose tightens on terror group. *CNN.* https://edition.cnn.com/2017/07/17/middleeast/raqqa-isis-brides/index.html

Peake, G., Gormley-Heenan, C., and Fitzduff, M. (2004) *From warlords to peacelords: Local leadership capacity in peace processes.* Jordanstown, Northern Ireland: INCORE.

Pemberton, A. and Aarten, P.G.M. (2018) Narrative in the study of victimological processes in terrorism and political violence: An initial exploration. *Studies in Conflict & Terrorism,* 41(7), 541–556.

Peracha, F.N., Khan, R.R., and Savage, S. (2016) Sabaoon: Education methods successfully countering and preventing violent extremism. In S. Zeiger (ed.), *Expanding research on countering violent extremism* (pp. 85–104). Abu Dhabi: Hedayah and Edith Cowan University.

Perera-W.A., H. (2016) The effects of memory conformity and the cross-race effect in eyewitness testimony. *SSRN Electronic Journal,* 2732189. https://papers.ssrn.com/sol3/papers.cfm?abstract_id=2732189

Perešin, A. (2015) Fatal attraction: Western muslimas and ISIS. *Perspectives on Terrorism,* 9(3). http://www.terrorismanalysts.com/pt/index.php/pot/article/view/427/html

Perloff, R.M. (2015) A three-decade retrospective on the hostile media effect. *Mass Communication and Society,* 18(6), 701–729.

Peterson, S., Reina, C.S., Waldman, D., and Becker, W.J. (2015) Using physiological methods to study emotions in organizations. *Research on Emotion in Organizations,* 11, 1–27.

Pew Research Center (2012, December 18) The global religious landscape. https://www.pewforum.org/2012/12/18/global-religious-landscape-exec/

Phelps, E.A., O'Connor, K.J., Cunningham, W.A., Funayma, E.S., Gatenby, J.C., Gore, J.C., and Banaji, M.R. (2000) Performance on indirect measures of race evaluation predicts amygdala activity. *Journal of Cognitive Neuroscience,* 12(5), 729–738.

Pillai, R. (1996) Crisis and the emergence of charismatic leadership in groups: An experimental investigation. *Journal of Applied Social Psychology,* 26(6), 543–562.

Pinker, S. (2002) *The blank slate: The modern denial of human nature.* New York: Penguin.

Pinker, S. (2012) *The better angels of our nature: Why violence has declined.* New York: Viking.

Popper, M. (2012) *Fact and fantasy about leadership.* Cheltenham, UK: Edward Elgar.

Post, J. (2004) *Leaders and their followers in a dangerous world: The psychology of political behavior.* Ithaca, NY: Cornell University Press.

Poulin, M., Holman, A., and Buffone, A. (2012) The neurogenetics of nice: Receptor genes for oxytocin and vasopressin interact with threat to predict prosocial behaviour. *Psychological Science,* 23(5), 446–452.

Prasad, D.Y.J. (2015) *A perspective on the Naxalite insurgency in Jharkhand and Bihar: Going beyond the grievance argument* (MA thesis, University of British Columbia, Vancouver). https://open.library.ubc.ca/cIRcle/collections/ubctheses/24/items/1.0165830

Press Trust of India (2014, November 5) Indian peace keeping force raped Tamil women during LTTE war: Lankan minister. *News 18.* https://www.news18.com/news/india/indian-peace-keeping-force-raped-tamil-women-during-ltte-war-lankan-minister-724149.html

Psaltis, C. (2016) Collective memory, social representations of intercommunal relations, and conflict transformation in divided Cyprus. *Peace and Conflict,* 22(1), 19–27.

Putnam, R. (2000) *Bowling alone: The collapse and revival of American community*. New York: Simon & Schuster.

Radovanović, B. (2019) Altruism in behavioural, motivational and evolutionary sense. *Filozofija i drustvo*, 30(1), 122–134.

Radsch, C.C. (2016) Media development and countering violent extremism: An uneasy relationship, a need for dialogue. *Center for International Media Assistance, National Endowment for Democracy.* https://www.cima.ned.org/wp-content/uploads/2016/10/CIMA-CVE-Paper_web-150ppi.pdf

Raffy, S. (2004) *Castro, el desleal*. Madrid: Santillana Ediciones.

Rand, D.G., Dreber, A., Ellingsen, T., Fudenberg, D., and Nowak, M.A. (2009) Positive interactions promote public cooperation. *Science*, 325(5945), 1272–1275.

Rand, D.G., Greene, J.D., and Nowak, M.A. (2012) Spontaneous giving and calculated greed. *Nature*, 489, 427–430.

Ratner, K.G. and Amodio, D.M. (2012) Seeing "us vs. them": Minimal group effects on the neural encoding of faces. *Journal of Experimental Social Psychology*, 49(2), 298–301.

Re, D.E. and Rule, N.O. (2016) The big man has a big mouth: Mouth width correlates with perceived leadership ability and actual leadership performance. *Journal of Experimental Social Psychology*, 63, 86–93.

Reh, S., Van Quaquebeke, N., and Giessner, S.R. (2017) The aura of charisma: A review on the embodiment perspective as signalling. *Leadership Quarterly*, 28(4), 486–507.

Rendell, L., Fogarty, L., Hoppitt, W.J.E., Morgan, T., Webster, M.M., and Laland, K.N. (2011) Cognitive culture: Theoretical and empirical insights into social learning strategies. *Trends in Cognitive Sciences*, 15(2), 68–76.

Reuter, M., Frenzel, C., Walter, N.T., Markett, S., and Montag, C. (2011) Investigating the genetic basis of altruism: The role of the COMT Val158Met polymorphism. *Social Cognitive and Affective Neuroscience*, 6(5), 662–668.

Richerson, P.J. and Boyd, R. (2005) *Not by genes alone: How culture transformed human evolution*. Chicago: University of Chicago Press.

Ricoeur, P. (2006) Memory—forgetting—history. In J. Rüsen (ed.), *Meaning and Representation in History*. Oxford: Berghahn Books.

Rock, D. (2009) *Your brain at work: Strategies for overcoming distraction, regaining focus, and working smarter all day long*. New York: HarperCollins.

Rock, D. (2016, November 7) Why we select toxic leaders. *Psychology Today*. https://www.psychologytoday.com/gb/blog/your-brain-work/201611/why-we-select-toxic-leaders

Rogers, P. (1995) Kill thy neighbor. *People*, 44(25). https://people.com/archive/kill-thy-neighbor-vol-44-no-25

Romano, C. (2013, March 18) Reason, emotion, and Hitler. *Chronicle of Higher Education*. https://www.chronicle.com/article/Reason-EmotionHitler/137883

Ronquillo, J., Denson, T.F., Lickel, B., Lu, Z.-L., Nandy, A., and Maddox, K.B. (2007) The effects of skin tone on race-related amygdala activity: An fMRI investigation. *Social Cognitive and Affective Neuroscience*, 2(1), 39–44.

Ross, G. (2011) *Who watches the watchmen? The conflict between national security and freedom of the press*. Washington, DC: National Intelligence University.

Ross, K. (2017) *Youth encounter programs in Israel: Pedagogy, identity, and social change*. Syracuse, NY: Syracuse University Press.

Ross, L. (1977) The intuitive psychologist and his shortcomings: Distortions in the attribution process. In L. Berkowitz (ed.), *Advances in experimental social psychology* (Vol. 10, pp. 173–220). New York: Academic Press.

Rotter, J.B. (1966) Generalized expectancies for internal versus external control of reinforcement. *Psychological Monographs: General and Applied*, 80(1), 1–28.

Roy, O. (2017, April 13) Who are the new jihadis? *The Guardian*. https://www.theguardian.com/news/2017/apr/13/who-are-the-new-jihadis

Rubin, R.D., Watson, P.D., Duff, M.C., and Cohen, N.J. (2014) The role of the hippocampus in flexible cognition and social behavior. *Frontiers in Human Neuroscience*, 8, 742. https://doi.org/10.3389/fnhum.2014.00742/full

Runciman, D. (2012, March 14) *The Righteous Mind* by Jonathan Haidt (review). *The Guardian*. https://www.theguardian.com/books/2012/mar/14/the-righteous-mind-jonathan-haidt-review

Rushton, J.P. (2004) Genetic and environmental contributions to pro-social attitudes: A twin study of social responsibility. *Proceedings, Biological Sciences*, 271(1557), 2583–2585.

Ryan, J.T., Hayes, P.A., and Craig, J.M. (2019) Leadership evolution for planetary health: A genomics perspective. *Challenges*, 10(1), 4.

Saad, G. and Greengross, G. (2014) Using evolutionary theory to enhance the brain imaging paradigm. *Frontiers in Human Neuroscience*. https://doi.org/10.3389/fnhum.2014.00452/full

Sageman, M. (2004) *Understanding terror networks*. Philadelphia: University of Pennsylvania Press.

Sapolsky, R.M. (2017) *Behave: The biology of humans at our best and worst*. New York: Penguin Random House.

Scaruffi, P. (2009) Wars and casualties of the 20th and 21st centuries. https://www.scaruffi.com/politics/massacre.html

Schacter, D.L., Guerin, S.A., and St Jacques, P.L. (2011) Memory distortion: An adaptive perspective. *Trends in Cognitive Sciences*, 15(10), 467–474.

Schaller, M., Simpson, J.A., and Kenrick, D.T. (eds.) (2014) *Evolution and social psychology*. New York: Psychology Press.

Schiffer, I. (1973) *Charisma: A psychoanalytic look at mass society*. Toronto: University of Toronto Press.

Schiller, D., Kanen, J.W., LeDoux, J.E., Monfils, M.H., and Phelps, E.A. (2013) Extinction during reconsolidation of threat memory diminishes prefrontal cortex involvement. *Proceedings of the National Academy of Sciences of the United States of America*, 110(50), 20040–20045.

Schreiber, D., Fonzo, G., Simmons, A.N., Dawes, C.T., Flagan, T., Fowler, J.H., and Paulus, M.P. (2013) Red brain, blue brain: Evaluative processes differ in Democrats and Republicans. *PLoS One*, 8(2), e52970.

Schulte-Rüther, M., Markowitsch, H.J., Shah, N.J., Fink, G.R., and Piefke, M. (2008) Gender differences in brain networks supporting empathy. *NeuroImage*, 42(1), 393–403.

Scott, E. (2020, February 22) All about catecholamines in the stress response: Fight or flight chemical messengers. *VeryWellMind*. https://www.verywellmind.com/all-about-catecholamines-3145098

Selimbeyoglu, A. and Parvizi, J. (2010) Electrical stimulation of the human brain: Perceptual and behavioral phenomena reported in the old and new literature. *Frontiers in Human Neuroscience*. https://doi.org/10.3389/fnhum.2010.00046/full

Settle, J.E., Dawes, C.T., Christakis, N.A., and Fowler, J.H. (2010) Friendships moderate an association between a dopamine gene variant and political ideology. *Journal of Politics*, 72(4), 1189–1198.

Shah, D.V., Hanna, A., and Bucy, E.P. (2015) Power of television images in a social media age: Linking biobehavioral and computational approaches via the second screen. *Annals of the American Academy of Political and Social Science*, 659(1), 225–245.

Shamir, B., Arthur, M.B., and House, R.J. (1994) The rhetoric of charismatic leadership: A theoretical extension, a case study, and implications for research. *Leadership Quarterly*, 5(1), 25–42.

Shamir, B., House, R.J., and Arthur, M.B. (1993) The motivational effects of charismatic leadership: A self-concept based theory. *Organization Science*, 4(4), 577–594.

Sharot, T., Shiner, T., Brown, A.C., Fan, J., and Dolan, R.J. (2009) Dopamine enhances expectation of pleasure in humans. *Current Biology*, 19(24), 2077–2080.

Sheng, F., Liu, Y., Zhou, B., Zhou, W., and Han, S. (2013) Oxytocin modulates the racial bias in neural responses to others' suffering. *Biological Psychology*, 92(2), 380–386.

Sherif, M., Harvey, O.J., White, B.J., Hood, W.R., and Sherif, C.W. (1961) *Intergroup conflict and cooperation: The Robbers Cave experiment*. Norman: Oklahoma University Press.

Sherman, L.E., Hernandez, L.M., Greenfield, P.M., and Dapretto, M. (2018) What the brain "likes": neural correlates of providing feedback on social media. *Social Cognitive and Affective Neuroscience*, 13(7), 699–707.

Sherman, L.E., Payton, A.A., Hernandez, L.M., Greenfield, P.M., and Dapretto, M. (2016) The power of the like in adolescence: Effects of peer influence on neural and behavioral responses to social media. *Psychological Science*, 27(7), 1027–1035.

Sherwood, H., Laville, S., Willsher, K., Knight, B., French, M., and Gambino, L. (2014, September 29) Schoolgirl jihadis: The female Islamists leaving home to join Isis fighters, *The Guardian*. https://www.theguardian.com/world/2014/sep/29/schoolgirl-jihadis-female-islamists-leaving-home-join-isis-iraq-syria

Shirky, C. (2009) *Here comes everybody: The power of organizing without organizations*. London: Penguin.

Shondrick, S.J. and Lord, Robert G. (2010) Implicit leadership and followership theories: Dynamic structures for leadership perceptions, memory, leader–follower processes. In G.P. Hodgkinson and J.K. Ford (eds.), *International review of industrial and organizational psychology* (Vol. 25). New York: Wiley.

Sillars, A. and Parry, D. (1982) Stress, cognition, and communication in interpersonal conflicts. *Communication Research*, 9(2), 201–226.

Silva, J.A., Derecho, D.V., Leong, G.B., Weinstock, R., and Ferrari, M.M. (2001) A classification of psychological factors leading to violent behaviour in posttraumatic stress disorder. *Journal of Forensic Sciences*, 31, 81–83.

Singer, P.W. and Brooking, E.T. (2018) *LikeWar: The weaponization of social media*. New York: Eamon Dolan/Houghton Mifflin Harcourt.

Slovic, P. (1987) Perception of risk. *Science*, 236(4799), 280–285.

Smith, C.O., Levine, D.W., Smith, E.P., Dumas, J., and Prinz, R.J. (2009) A developmental perspective of the relationship of racial–ethnic identity to self-construct, achievement, and behavior in African American children. *Cultural Diversity and Ethnic Minority Psychology*, 15(2), 145–157.

Smith, D. (2013, December 8) Francois Pienaar: "When the whistle blew, South Africa changed forever." *The Guardian*. https://www.theguardian.com/world/2013/dec/08/nelson-mandela-francois-pienaar-rugby-world-cup

Smith, K. (2020, January 2) 258 incredible and interesting Twitter stats and statistics. *Brandwatch*. https://www.brandwatch.com/blog/twitter-stats-and-statistics/

Smith, R. (2005) *The utility of force: The art of war in the modern world*. London: Vintage.

Soon, C.S., Brass, M., Heinze, H., and Haynes, J. (2008) Unconscious determinants of free decisions in the human brain. *Nature Neuroscience*, 11(5), 543–545.

Southern Poverty Law Center (2019) Groups. https://www.splcenter.org/fighting-hate/extremist-files/groups

Spencer-Oatey, H. (2012) What is culture? A compilation of quotations. *GlobalPAD Core Concepts*. http://www.warwick.ac.uk/globalpadintercultural

Spisak, B.R., Blaker, N.M., Lefevre, C.E., Moore, F.R., and Krebbers, K.F.B. (2014) A face for all seasons: Searching for context-specific leadership traits and discovering a general preference for perceived health. *Frontiers in Human Neuroscience*, 8, 792. https://doi.org/10.3389/fnhum.2014.00792/full

Stallen, M. and Sanfey, A.G. (2013) The cooperative brain. *The Neuroscientist*, 19(3), 292–303.

Statista (2020) Global digital population as of January 2020. https://www.statista.com/statistics/617136/digital-population-worldwide/

Staub, E. (1989) *The roots of evil: The origins of genocide and other group violence*. New York: Cambridge University Press.

Steinberg, L. (2008) A social neuroscience perspective on adolescent risk-taking. *Developmental Review*, 28(1), 78–106.

Stewart, F. (ed.) (2008) *Horizontal inequalities and conflict: Understanding group violence in multiethnic societies*. Basingstoke, UK: Palgrave Macmillan.

Stewart, P., Waller, B., and Schubert, J. (2009) Presidential speechmaking style: Emotional response to micro-expressions of facial affect. *Motivation and Emotion*, 33(2), 125–135.

Stone, A. (2007, September 12) Most think founders wanted Christian USA. *USA Today*.

Suedfeld, P., Leighton, D., and Conway, L.G. (2006) Integrative complexity and decisionmaking in international confrontations. In M. Fitzduff and C.E. Stout (eds.), *The psychology of resolving global conflicts: From war to peace* (pp. 211–238). Westport, CT: Praeger.

Suedfeld, P. and Schaller, M. (2002) Authoritarianism and the Holocaust: Some cognitive and affective implications. In L.S. Newman and R. Erber (eds.), *Understanding genocide: The social psychology of the Holocaust*. Oxford: Oxford University Press.

Sullivan, M. (2016, March 18) Your brain might be hard-wired for altruism. *UCLA Newsroom*. http://newsroom.ucla.edu/releases/your-brain-might-be-hard-wired-for-altruism

Sunstein, C.R. (1996) *Social norms and social roles*. Working Paper No. 36. Chicago: Coase-Sandor Institute for Law & Economics.

Svetlova, M., Nichols, S.R., and Brownell, C.A. (2010) Toddlers' prosocial behavior: From instrumental to empathic to altruistic helping. *Child Development*, 81(6), 1814–1827.

Swaine, J. (2018, January 20) Twitter admits far more Russian bots posted on election than it had disclosed. *The Guardian*. https://www.theguardian.com/technology/2018/jan/19/twitter-admits-far-more-russian-bots-posted-on-election-than-it-had-disclosed

Taber, C.S. and Young, E. (2013) Political information processing. In L. Huddy, D.O. Sears, and J.S. Levy (eds.), *The Oxford Handbook of Political Psychology* (2nd ed.). Oxford: Oxford University Press.

Tabibnia, G. and Lieberman, M.D. (2007) Fairness and cooperation are rewarding: Evidence from social cognitive neuroscience. *Annals of the New York Academy of Sciences*, 1118, 90–101.

Tactical Tech (2018) *Tools of the influence industry*. https://ourdataourselves.tacticaltech.org/posts/methods-and-practices/

Tajfel, H. (1978) Interindividual and intergroup behaviour. In H. Tajfel (ed.), *Differentiation between groups: Studies in the social psychology of intergroup relations* (pp. 27–60). London: Academic Press.

Takeuchi, S. and Marara, J. (2009) *Conflict and land tenure in Rwanda*. Tokyo: JICA Research Institute.

Tetlock, P.E., Kristel, O.V., Elson, S.B., Green, M.C., and Lerner J.S. (2000) The psychology of the unthinkable: Taboo trade-offs, forbidden base rates, and heretical counterfactuals. *Journal of Personality and Social Psychology*, 78(5), 853–870.

Theodoridis, A.G. and Nelson, A.J. (2012) Of BOLD claims and excessive fears: A call for caution and patience regarding political neuroscience. *Political Psychology*, 33(1), 27–43.

Thornhill, R. and Fincher, C.L. (2014) The parasite-stress theory of sociality, the behavioral immune system, and human social and cognitive uniqueness. *Evolutionary Behavioral Sciences*, 8(4), 257–264.

Tiemessen, A.E. (2004) After Arusha: Gacaca justice in post-genocide Rwanda. *African Studies Quarterly*, 8(1), 57–76.

Tigue, C., Borak, D., O'Connor, J., Schandl, C., and Feinberg, D. (2011) Voice pitch influences voting behavior. *Evolution and Human Behavior*, 33(3), 210–216.

Tiihonen, J., Rautiainen, M., Ollila, H., Repo-Tiihonen, E., Virkkunen, M., Palotie, A., Pietiläinen, O., Kristiansson, K., Joukamaa, M., Lauerma, H., Saarela, J., Tyni, S., Vartiainen, H., Paananen, J., Goldman, D., and Paunio, T. (2015) Genetic background of extreme violent behavior. *Molecular Psychiatry*, 20, 786–792.

Tomasello, M. and Hamann, K. (2012) Collaboration in young children. *Quarterly Journal of Experimental Psychology*, 65(1), 1–12.

Tomasello, M., Melis, A.P., Tennie, C., Wyman, E., and Herrmann, E. (2012) Two key steps in the evolution of human cooperation. *Current Anthropology*, 53(6), 673–692.

Tony Blair Institute for Global Change (2018) *Global Extremism Monitor 2017: Violent Islamist extremism in 2017*. London: Tony Blair Institute for Global Change.

Tooby, J. and Cosmides, L. (1990) The past explains the present: Emotional adaptations and the structure of ancestral environments. *Ethology and Sociobiology*, 11(4–5), 375–424.

Travis, A. (2008, August 20) MI5 report challenges views on terrorism in Britain. *The Guardian*. https://www.theguardian.com/uk/2008/aug/20/uksecurity.terrorism1

Triandis, H., Bontempo, R., Villareal, M., Asai, M., and Lucca, N. (1988) Individualism and collectivism: Cross-cultural perspectives on self–ingroup relationship. *Journal of Personality and Social Psychology*, 54(2), 323–338.

Truskanov, N. and Prat, Y. (2018) Cultural transmission in an ever-changing world: Trial-and-error copying may be more robust than precise imitation. *Philosophical Transactions of the Royal Society B: Biological Sciences*, 373(1743). https://doi.org/10.1098/rstb.2017.0050

Tskhay, K.O., Xu, H., and Rule, N.O. (2014) Perceptions of leadership success from nonverbal cues communicated by orchestra conductors. *Leadership Quarterly*, 25(5), 901–911.

Tusche, A., Kahnt, T., Wisniewski, D., and Haynes, J.D. (2013) Automatic processing of political preferences in the human brain. *NeuroImage*, 72, 174–182.

Tversky, A. and Kahneman, D. (1974) Judgment under uncertainty: Heuristics and biases. *Science*, 185, 1124–1131.

Twenge, J.M., Baumeister, R.F., DeWall, C.N., Ciarocco, N.J., and Bartels, J.M. (2007) Social exclusion decreases prosocial behavior. *Journal of Personality and Social Psychology*, 92(1), 56–66.

Ulman, R.B. and Apse, D.W. (1983) The group psychology of mass madness: Jonestown. *Political Psychology*, 4, 637–661.

UN Women (2019) Facts and figures: Leadership and political participation. https://www.unwomen.org/en/what-we-do/leadership-and-political-participation/facts-and-figures

USAID (2009) *Religion, conflict and peacebuilding*. Washington, DC: USAID.

Vaidhyanathan, S. (2018) *Antisocial media: How Facebook disconnects us and undermines democracy*. Oxford: Oxford University Press.

Van Bavel, J.J. and Cunningham, W.A. (2009) Self-categorization with a novel mixed-race group moderates automatic social and racial biases. *Personality and Social Psychology Bulletin*, 35, 321–335.

Van Bavel, J.J., Earls, H., Morris, J., and Cunningham, W.A. (2013) *Identity tunes rapid person perception: Group membership overrides initial racial bias*. Unpublished manuscript.

van der Plas, E.A.A., Boes, A.D., Wemmie, J.A., Tranel, D., and Nopoulos, P. (2010) Amygdala volume correlates positively with fearfulness in normal healthy girls. *Social Cognitive and Affective Neuroscience*, 5(4), 424–431.

Van Hiel, A, Onraet, E, and De Pauw, S. (2010) The relationship between social-cultural attitudes and behavioral measures of cognitive style: A meta-analytic integration of studies. *Journal of Personality*, 78(6), 1765–1799.

Van Vugt, M. and Ahuja, A. (2010) *Selected: Why some people lead, why others follow, and why it matters*. London: Profile Books.

Van Vugt, M. and Grabo, A.E. (2015) The many faces of leadership: An evolutionary-psychology approach. *Current Directions in Psychological Science*, 24(6), 484–489.

Van Vugt, M., Hogan, R., and Kaiser, R.B. (2008) Leadership, followership, and evolution: Some lessons from the past. *American Psychologist*, 63(3), 182–196.

Velton, R. (2017, April 25) The "silent killer" of Africa's albinos. *BBC Future*. https://www.bbc.com/future/article/20170425-the-silent-killer-of-africas-albinos

Verbaarschot, C., Haselager, P., and Farquhar, J. (2016) Detecting traces of consciousness in the process of intending to act. *Experimental Brain Research*, 234, 1945–1956.

Victoroff, J., Quota, S., Adelman, J., Celinska, B., Stern, N., Wilcox, R., and Sapolsky, R. (2011) Support for religio-political aggression among teenaged boys in Gaza: Part II: Neuroendocrinological findings. *Aggressive Behavior*, 37(2), 121–132.

Vignoles, V., Schwartz, S., and Luyckx, K. (2011) Introduction: Toward an integrative view of identity. In S.J. Schwartz, K. Luyckx, and V.L. Vignoles (eds.), *Handbook of identity theory and research* (pp. 1–27). Berlin: Springer Science + Business Media.

Volkan, V. (1998, August) *Transgenerational transmissions and chosen traumas: An element of large-group identity*. Opening address, XIII International Congress, International Association of Group Psychotherapy, London.

Volkan, V. (2001) Transgenerational transmissions and chosen traumas: An aspect of large-group identity. *Group Analysis*, 34(1), 79–97.

Volkan, V. (2004) *Blind trust: Large groups and their leaders in times of crisis and terror*. Durham, NC: Pitchstone.

Volkan, V. (2009) Large-group identity, international relations and psychoanalysis. *International Forum of Psychoanalysis*, 18(4), 206–213.

Volman, I., von Borries, A.K.L., Bulten, B.H., Verkes, R.J., Toni, I., and Roelofs, K. (2016) Testosterone modulates altered prefrontal control of emotional actions in psychopathic offenders. *eNeuro*, 3(1), 1–9.

Vosoughi, S., Roy, D., and Aral, S. (2018) The spread of true and false news online. *Science*, 359(6380), 1146–1151.

Wade, L. (2011, January 28) Irish apes: Tactics of de-humanization. *The Society Pages*. https://thesocietypages.org/socimages/2011/01/28/irish-apes-tactics-of-de-humanization/

Waldman, D., Balthazard, P.A., and Peterson, S. (2011) Social cognitive neuroscience and leadership. *Leadership Quarterly*, 22(6), 1092–1106.

Wall, K. and Choksi, M. (2018, May 22) A chance to rewrite history: The women fighters of the Tamil Tigers. *Longreads*. https://longreads.com/2018/05/22/a-chance-to-rewrite-history-the-women-fighters-of-the-tamil-tigers/

Waller, J. (2006) Becoming evil: How ordinary people commit genocide and mass killing. In M. Fitzduff and C.E. Stout (eds.), *The psychology of resolving global conflicts: From war to peace*. Westport, CT: Praeger.

Walsh, D, and Zway, A.S. (2018, September 4) A Facebook war: Libyans battle on the streets and on screens. *New York Times*. https://www.nytimes.com/2018/09/04/world/middleeast/libya-facebook.html

Walsh, K. (2001) Collective amnesia and the mediation of painful pasts: The representation of France in the Second World War. *International Journal of Heritage Studies*, 7(1), 83–98.

Walsh, K., Uddin, M., Soliven, R., Wildman, D., and Bradley, B. (2014) Associations between the SS variant of 5-HTTLPR and PTSD among adults with histories of childhood emotional abuse: Results from two African American independent samples. *Journal of Affective Disorders*, 161, 91–96.

Walter, B. (2017) The new new civil wars. *Annual Review of Political Science*, 20, 469–486.

Warneken, F. and Tomasello, M. (2010) Helping and cooperation at 14 months of age. *Infancy*, 11(3), 271–294.

Webber, D., Chernikova, M., Kruglanski, A., Gelfand, M., Hettiarachchi, M., Gunaratna, R., Lafreniere, M.-A., and Bélanger, J. (2018) Deradicalizing detained terrorists. *Political Psychology*, 39(3), 539–556.

Weierter, S. (1997) Who wants to play "follow the leader?" A theory of charismatic relationships based on routinized charisma and follower characteristics. *Leadership Quarterly*, 8, 171–193.

Weinberg, L. and Eubank, W. (2011) Women's involvement in terrorism. *Gender Issues*, 28(1–2), 22–49.

Weinschenk, S. (2012, September 11) Why we're all addicted to texts, Twitter and Google. *Psychology Today*. https://www.psychologytoday.com/ca/blog/brain-wise/201209/why-were-all-addicted-texts-twitter-and-google?collection=157448

Weir, K. (2017) Why we believe alternative facts: How motivation, identity and ideology combine to undermine human judgment. *Monitor on Psychology*, 48(5). https://www.apa.org/monitor/2017/05/alternative-facts

Weiss, K.M. and Buchanan, A.V. (2009) *The mermaid's tale: Four billion years of cooperation in the making of living things*. Cambridge, MA: Harvard University Press.

Westen, D. (2008) *The political brain: The role of emotion in deciding the fate of the nation*. New York: PublicAffairs.

Westen, D., Blagov, P.S., Harenski, K., Kilts, C., and Hamann, S. (2006) Neural bases of motivated reasoning: An fMRI Study of emotional constraints on partisan political judgment in the 2004 U.S. presidential election. *Journal of Cognitive Neuroscience*, 18(11), 1947–1958.

Whicker, M.L. (1996) *Toxic leaders: When organizations go bad*. Westport, CT: Quorum Books.

White, R.F. (2017) Political behavior and biology: Evolutionary leadership and followership. In S.A. Peterson and A. Somit (eds.), *Handbook of biology and politics* (pp. 22–49). Cheltenham, UK: Edward Elgar.

Why Boko Haram uses female suicide-bombers. (2017, 23 October). *The Economist*.

Wilde, R. (2018) Who were Hitler's supporters? Who backed the Führer and why. *ThoughtCo*. https://www.thoughtco.com/who-supported-hitler-and-why-1221371

Willis, J. and Todorov, A. (2006) First impressions: Making up your mind after a 100-ms exposure to a face. *Psychological Science*, 17(7), 592–598.

Wilson, J. (2000, November 18) How the real IRA recruits boys into a life of terrorism. *The Guardian*. https://www.theguardian.com/uk/2000/nov/18/northernireland.uksecurity

Winter, C. (2017) *Media jihad: The Islamic State's doctrine for information warfare*. London: International Centre for the Study of Radicalisation and Political Violence.

Wolpert, S. (2016, May 31) The teenage brain on social media. *UCLA Newsroom*. https://newsroom.ucla.edu/releases/the-teenage-brain-on-social-media

Wrangham, R. and Peterson, D. 1996. *Demonic males: Apes and the origins of human violence*. Boston: Houghton Mifflin.

Wright, R. (1999) *Nonzero: The logic of human destiny*. New York: Pantheon.

Xu, X., Zuo, X., Wang, X., and Han S. (2009) Do you feel my pain? Racial group membership modulates empathic neural responses. *Journal of Neuroscience*, 29(26), 8525–8529.

Yamagishi, T. and Mifune, N. (2016) Parochial altruism: Does it explain modern human group psychology? *Current Opinion in Psychology*, 7, 39–41.

Yang, H.-P., Wang, L., Han, L., and Wang, S.C. (2013) Nonsocial functions of hypothalamic oxytocin. *International Scholarly Research Notices*, 179272.

Yapp, R. (2016, December 9) The toxic triangle—the environment and followers of toxic leaders. *Leadership Forces*. https://www.leadershipforces.com/toxic-leadership-environment-followers/

Yeomans, R. (2005) Cults of death and fantasies of annihilation: The Croatian Ustasha movement in power, 1941–45. *Central Europe*, 3(2), 121–142.

Youngblood, S. (2017) What is peace journalism? *Media and Peace Building Research Project*. https://mediapeaceproject.smpa.gwu.edu/2017/12/14/what-is-peace-journalism/

Zaki, J., López, G., and Mitchell, J.P. (2014) Activity in ventromedial prefrontal cortex co-varies with revealed social preferences: Evidence for person-invariant value. *Social Cognitive and Affective Neuroscience*, 9(4), 464–469.

Zambakari, C. (2017, February 16) Challenges of liberal peace and statebuilding in divided societies. *Accord*. https://www.accord.org.za/conflict-trends/challenges-liberal-peace-statebuilding-divided-societies/

Zamboni, G., Gozzi, M., Krueger, F., Duhamel, J.R., Sirigu, A., and Grafman, J. (2009) Individualism, conservatism, and radicalism as criteria for processing political beliefs: A parametric fMRI study. *Social Neuroscience*, 4(5), 367–383.

Zephoria (2019) The top 20 valuable Facebook statistics. https://zephoria.com/top-15-valuable-facebook-statistics/

Zhang, T.-Y. and Meaney, M.J. (2010) Epigenetics and the environmental regulation of the genome and its function. *Annual Review of Psychology*, 61, 439–466.

Zimbardo, P.G., Haney, C., Banks, W.C., and Jaffe, D. (1973) *The psychology of imprisonment: Privation, power and pathology*. Unpublished manuscript.

Zoria, Y. (2020) Baltic "elves" launch online database of pro-Russian trolls to tackle propaganda. *Euromaidan Press*. http://euromaidanpress.com/2018/01/20/baltic-elves-launch-vatnikas-online-database-of-pro-russian-trolls-to-tackle-propaganda/

Index

For the benefit of digital users, indexed terms that span two pages (e.g., 52–53) may, on occasion, appear on only one of those pages.

Printed in the USA
CPSIA information can be obtained
at www.ICGtesting.com
CBHW081437240124
3715CB00003BA/10